THE MENTAL VACCINE FOR COVID-19

Praise for *The Mental Vaccine for COVID-19*

'Raj Persaud's original and inventive take on the mental health impact of the Covid19 pandemic will shock and inform you in equal measures.'

Professor Dr Robert Howard,
University College London Division of Psychiatry

'This book messed up my entire day. I had planned to skim through it, then maybe read a few chapters. But right from the beginning I was hooked. I read, and even at times re-read, all the chapters in one sitting. And may do so again.

There are three reasons why this is such a compelling book. First, it is very well written by a psychiatrist with lots of media experience. It is fast-paced and compelling because the author wants and needs to cover a lot of ground. The book has case studies, personal stories and complex ideas explained very clearly.

Second the book is strongly evidence-based; it is packed with detailed, up-to-date references to academic papers and books in a wide range of areas. The author is a polymath, with degrees and experience in many areas of research. It cuts through the Gordian knot of academic complexity and jargon and makes the results of scientifically executed papers easily accessible.

Third, and perhaps most importantly, is the author's insight. Raj is no ordinary psychiatrist interested in subtle diagnoses; he is interested in what works and why in the messy and complex area of human affairs. He is not afraid to take on the establishment and slaughter some of the shibboleths around the COVID-19 crisis. This takes confidence and courage, and is the result of a lot of academic reading, client contact and clear thinking.

The book has written in response to the current crisis, but has the wisdom of the ages.'

Professor Adrian Furnham,
University College London Division of Psychology and Language Sciences

THE MENTAL VACCINE FOR COVID-19

COPING WITH CORONA
A GUIDE TO PANDEMIC PSYCHOLOGY

Dr Raj Persaud FRCPsych

AMBERLEY

Cover image inside the virus symbol comes from a wood engraving entitled 'Mrs Aesop', kindly donated by Hilary Paynter, all rights reserved. She is one of the UK's leading wood engravers and Past President of the Royal Society of Painter-Printmakers. www.hilarypaynter.com

First published 2021

Amberley Publishing
The Hill, Stroud
Gloucestershire, GL5 4EP

www.amberley-books.com

Copyright © Raj Persaud, 2021

The right of Raj Persaud to be identified as the Author of this work has been asserted in accordance with the Copyright, Designs and Patents Act 1988.

ISBN 978 1 3981 1049 6 (hardback)
ISBN 978 1 3981 1050 2 (ebook)

British Library Cataloguing in Publication Data. A catalogue record for this book is available from the British Library.

1 2 3 4 5 6 7 8 9 10

Typesetting by SJmagic DESIGN SERVICES, India.
Printed in the UK.

'Between two evils, I always pick the one I never tried before.'

Mae West

'Men get the war they deserve.'

Jean-Paul Sartre

'When you come to a fork in the road, take it.'

Yogi Berra

In memory of Dr Peter Bruggen (1934–2018), a teacher and then a friend, who collaborated in many of the ideas and some of the excerpts that follow, revealing to me how much more there is to psychiatry than doctors realise.

Author royalties from the sale of this book are being donated to the Association for Post-Natal Illness (www.apni.org) and the new charity Silver Stories (www.silverstories.co.uk).

The APNI provides support to mothers suffering from post-natal illness, increases public awareness of the illness and encourages research into its cause. Dr Raj Persaud is a Trustee. Most people today have heard the term 'baby blues' used to describe a mild, short period of depression which many women experience after childbirth. Fewer people are aware that as many as 10 per cent of all recently delivered women develop postnatal depression, which is much more serious and debilitating, and could have long-term effects on mother and baby. Indeed, statistically speaking, the chances of developing a major mental illness, for any woman, appear highest in the period shortly after childbirth.

Silver Stories is based in Cornwall; it's a wonderfully simple idea. Young readers (Silver Readers) who are children in primary or secondary school telephone older people (Silver Listeners) residing in care homes, or living on their own, and read aloud to them every week. They laugh together with the Silver Listeners, sing together, and lift each other's spirits. It gives older people the contact they love with children, and it gives the children confidence as readers, and the knowledge that they are making someone really happy. The charity is the brainchild of married couple Elisabeth and David Carney Haworth; he is a retired police officer and she is a retired primary school head teacher. They received an honour for their idea. Dame Esther Rantzen, a Trustee, suggested the author donate the royalties to this charity.

CONTENTS

TO THE READER

At various points in the following narrative, self-destructive acts of those negatively affected by the pandemic are described in explicit detail.

Don't read on if you're of a very nervous disposition.

There is controversy over whether such graphic accounts might also encourage readers to self-harm. But these pages intend to deliver a shot of hope. They inject resilience, no matter how terrible you feel. The impact of the contagion on happiness can be resisted successfully, as comprehensively set out for the first time in this guide. This virus has been messing with our minds, as well as our bodies.

If you're just too low, or emotional, right now, please also reach out. There are organisations and charities devoted to these predicaments. Worldwide, the best known might be the Samaritans,[1] whom I have supported in various capacities.

Be warned: I don't shy away from hard-hitting depictions of the havoc this epidemic has wreaked on our emotional health. We delve into personal stories – some despairing, many inspiring. Be on guard, because I don't pull any punches.

PREFACE

WHY A MENTAL VACCINE?

Press coverage of the penultimate day of one of the worst years of modern times, 2020, was constrained by the challenge of finding anything encouraging to say.

However, Prince Harry and Meghan, the Duke and Duchess of Sussex, used the first podcast they recorded for Spotify to reflect on difficulties faced by many during the pandemic. Journalists were grateful for a positive story in the midst of the horror.[1] After all, it was earlier in 2020 that Prince Harry had talked for the first time about being in therapy. Maybe some tips on mental health and well-being might be forthcoming from this new podcast series, reputed to have cost Spotify £18 million?

Celebrity pals, including Sir Elton John and James Corden, as well as Brené Brown, described by the press as the 'world's biggest self-help guru', and Deepak Chopra, the renowned spiritual healer, joined a host of luminaries sharing what they now understood better about themselves: what gives them hope in the darkness.

Some talked, impressively, about how they had helped many less fortunate than themselves in practical ways. In the 30-minute 'holiday special', recorded at the Californian mansion Meghan and Prince Harry acquired in June, the Duchess ended the show with these words of comfort: 'From us I'll say no matter what life throws at you guys, trust us when we say, love wins.' The Duke endorsed the sentiment, adding: 'Love always wins.'

This is typical of the sort of comforting recommended by the media throughout the year. It's a touching sentiment. But is it fundamentally helpful to anyone experiencing emotional turmoil as a result of the pandemic?

I don't want to pick on Prince Harry and Meghan in particular, who seem to be well-meaning, but it was this kind of platitude that inspired me, or perhaps irritated me, into producing this guide.

And then came 'that' interview in March 2021 where Meghan confessed to Oprah Winfrey her frightening suicidal thoughts. The juxtaposition of the sentiments in the first podcast – 'love always wins' – with the dark place Meghan eventually appeared to have spiralled down to prompted an inevitable question: was 'love always wins' really the answer to suicidal depression? It is one of the crucial questions of our time, and I hope to finally settle that debate, and others, in this guide.

A mental vaccine for COVID-19.

Over and over again I found myself disturbed by official or popular guidance on staying resilient. It ranged from boring and repetitive to unimaginative and ill-informed, and I couldn't figure out how it was supposed to have any pragmatic meaning for anyone. Instructions being peddled included tired old pop psychology, and there was no real acknowledgement that this was a completely different scale and type of distress than anything the planet had ever faced before.

Another problem was that the counsel being dispensed through the media often hid an agenda which said more about the advisor than about the quality of the advice. For example, it felt a bit like Prince Harry and Meghan were casting themselves in some kind of latter-day *Romeo and Juliet* intrigue. The true love of the young couple was up against opposing forces from the disapproving parents, as in Shakespeare's tragedy.

Yet no matter how little these exhortations helped those confronting the pandemic, editors just kept peddling impassioned gushing. It was advice as entertainment; or was it the other way round? I got confused.

To be scrupulously fair to the 'ex-royals', they were by no means the only ones guilty of promulgating pointless prescriptions. Doctors were popping up on TV, dishing out mind medicine. The trouble was, for those on the inside of psychiatry, these all looked like the watery placebo arm of a vaccine trial.

It was designed to look and feel like the real thing. But it wasn't.

A practising NHS GP, columnist and broadcaster was one of those 'experts' dispensing advice on the BBC News website.[2] Her five mental health tips for lockdown included the following directive:

Work out what you are not in control of and write a list of those things down. Every time one of those things comes into your head recognise it as something you can't control and try to let go of it to maintain your emotional energy.

When I first heard this injunction, broadcast to the nation, I was alarmed. These directives aren't just useless, they could even be counterproductive; more a poison than a placebo. 'Try to let go of it' is akin to saying that when trying to feel better you should 'try to feel better'.

In terrible therapy, which is common, patients are constantly asked to make laundry lists. If anything might be a recipe for making you suicidal, this would be it. Another favourite in this realm of duping the patient into believing some pragmatic strategy is being offered is the 'keep a mood diary' ploy – under pandemic pressure this is likely, in my opinion, to drive you psychotic.

It is certainly true that intrusive, unhelpful thoughts[3] are a real problem in a pandemic. No disrespect is intended towards this particular BBC NHS family doctor; after all, GPs know a huge amount more medicine than I do, as a lowly consultant psychiatrist. But the absence of proper specialist emotional health expertise made available to the public has meant we've suffered an epidemic of abjectly poor advice. Mental health problems begin precisely at the point where everything that has 'cheered us up' before no longer works. And the pandemic puts us under immediate unprecedented pressure that could be life-altering in the same way as a major car crash. The stakes are high.

So, where are the pragmatic tips to help us feel fundamentally better? And why abandon cutting-edge neural science when disseminating resilience inoculation strategies?

A team led by Professor Marie Banich[4] used advanced brain scanning technology to reveal how to get rid of unwanted thoughts. The investigation involved marrying the latest machine-learning advances with ground-breaking neuroimaging.

The key finding is that before you can think clearly about something new,[5] you have to cease dwelling on the distracting apprehension you were worrying about before. If you don't, then a kind of brain fog descends, where the previous ruminations prevent you considering new or refreshing ideas or experiences.

Coronavirus has produced a sort of head haze because we find it difficult to stop ruminating about a whole host of qualms over new predicaments. In an exam-oriented culture, showing off intellectual ability, and in particular memory, seems paramount to success at work. At dinner parties, the requirement for witty repartee and the recall of arresting anecdotes means our brains primarily serve as vehicles of retention. But the authors of this study[3] argue that the ability to remove irrelevant or unhelpful information from mental space is also essential, particularly to emotional health. They could visualise on a brain scan the physical trace of neural activity representing an idea, and watch it fade in response to elimination efforts by the owner of those nerve cells. However, they could also witness the faint leftover trace of brain activity, signalling that the last misgiving you were trying to suppress still hadn't been fully dispatched. It was still lurking there, able to interfere with new ideas.

Deficits in this capability – to clear the mind – become a prominent feature of many psychiatric disorders including depression, generalized anxiety disorder, post-traumatic stress (PTSD), and obsessive-compulsive (OCD), all of which have become more prominent because of the pandemic.

Sherlock Holmes, perhaps literature's most famous proponent of a sharpened intelligence as a weapon against adversaries, declared that a mind is like an attic.[3] It can fill with clutter, rendering it difficult to retrieve resources when needed. Before long, you can't move about in your head space without tumbling over tat.

Sir Arthur Conan Doyle, the creator of Sherlock Holmes, was himself a doctor before becoming an author, and in the first book to feature the great detective, *A Study in Scarlet*, he has the mastermind declaring,

> The skilful workman is very careful indeed as to what he takes into his brain-attic. He will have nothing but the tools which may help him in doing his work ... It is of the highest importance, therefore, not to have useless facts elbowing out the useful ones.[3]

The pandemic represents a fabulous opportunity for a massive declutter, not just of your actual attic, but also of your unconscious.

Depression is characterised by intrusive negative thoughts and memories, anxiety by repetitive concerns about future adversities, obsessive-compulsive disorder by concerns over contamination.

Rumination lies at the heart of psychiatric disorder, particularly in the pandemic. That negativity doesn't just hijack our lives for a significant period of time; the obsessing also disturbs any newly arriving thoughts, so they invariably become deflected as well. Musing that goes nowhere, just in an aversive loop, imprisons us.

We think of the virus jailing us, through a variety of restrictions, or Boris Johnson throwing away the key, yet the toughest sentence we served was the way our minds fixated on unhelpful preoccupations. Our usual distractions that helped us maintain emotional control went south every time the Chief Scientific Officer took the stage to announce a new tier of restrictions. Going out and participating in fun and games or socialising played a vital role in our mental as well as physical health.

Obsessive-compulsive thinking causes distress through recurring thoughts such as, 'If I don't wash my hands yet again, I'll catch Covid.' In anxiety, the rumination might be, 'That person coughed over me, now I've got it.'

While sitting inside a brain imaging scanner, participants in this study[4] were told either to replace a thought (e.g. replace 'apple' with 'mountain'); clear all thoughts (akin to mindfulness meditation – become aware of your thoughts, and then distance yourself from ideas – attempt to clear your whole mind); or just directly suppress a particular thought (focus on it and then deliberately stop thinking about it).

The key finding from the study[5] by Professor Banich is that these contrasting mental strategies – 'replace', 'clear' or 'suppress' – produce different success rates. For the first time science could directly peer into your cerebral hemispheres and tell whether you really had forgotten something, as opposed to merely believing you had. The brain activity signature associated with any particular idea could be seen on the scanner to visibly fade at different rates, depending on the strategy deployed.

The researchers could literally read your mind.

But the nerve activity afterwards was different depending on whether the old thought was still there, though fading, indicating that to have new, fresh reflections you must completely get rid of the old ones. Forgetting, even if temporary, is vital to psychological change. Creating a new mood requires you to eliminate the old one conclusively.

The subjects taking part in this experiment often thought they had cleared their minds of a previous thought, yet the brain scanner revealed they hadn't completely. This lingering previous cogitation may explain why, despite our best efforts, we remain unable to improve our temper and move on. The old thought is still in there, influencing us, even when we believe it's gone.

To really declutter your mind, which is so vital at these times, you are going to need a really proper vigorous mental spring clean. In our clinic we call this 'clearing the attic', and this becomes a vital aspect of well-being in the face of adversity. How to achieve that?

As the study revealed, there are at least *three* distinct, relatively successful strategies for removing trouble from your mind: replace that apprehension with another idea, suppress that specific trepidation, or clear the mind of all thoughts.

The pandemic bestowed on you a host of losses and new fears, yet at the same time lockdown measures robbed you of all the normal ways of diverting yourself from rumination. You couldn't go and play tennis, shoot pool or hang out with friends – the myriad distractions which helped you disengage.

From a mental health standpoint, it was unprecedented. A perfect storm.

We shall discuss in more detail the particular strategies I have found most helpful in my clinical practice, informed by research, to weather this hurricane. Yet many survivors have intuitively grasped the central importance of this project, working out their own personal techniques.

Empty 'cheer-up' reassurances and 'love-always-wins' platitudes are not nearly decisive enough for individuals facing these terrible predicaments. Psychiatric problems begin precisely where 'cheer-up' advice fails. Obscure studies like Professor Banich's[4] are lifesaving.

In a pandemic, as in life, once you grasp the essential mental conundrum you should focus on, this immediately renders you more resilient.

I explore in this guide powerful psychological techniques which don't require medication, and which will help you to handle these worries. These originate from my thirty years of clinical practice and involvement with research. One strategy refers to a technique termed 'Worry Timetable' (see chapter 1). This is a practical method of postponing rumination. An ability to transition emotionally between being in the 'future', 'present' or 'past' is also part of the mental vaccine, and I will explain what that means later.

The key point is you need to become more aware of superior strategies for achieving better control of your individual mentality. A temporary fix simply won't work. The precise effectiveness of the various vaccines on offer, and in the pipeline, are statistics incessantly pored over in the media, so where is such concern for the effectiveness of the mental protections being offered?

Though they will be able to move freely after lockdown, so the difference won't be readily apparent, the mentally unvaccinated will, unfortunately, remain psychologically imprisoned by their short-term emotional straitjacket.

I present startling scientific evidence later, in Part 3, that the effects on our nerves from the current pandemic are liable to be much more enduring, even lasting for decades or possibly generations to come. The implication is that the mental vaccine is in fact more important than any jab in your arm.

Yet I'm not that surprised the family doctor used by the BBC for mental health advice[2] may not be aware of the latest neuroscience. No one should reasonably expect this otherwise perfectly competent BBC GP to be abreast of the specific scholarship in this area. Medicine and neuroscience are just too extensive as fields for any one physician to know everything about everything. And they are ever expanding. But the mental vaccines are out there, in the otherwise obscure academic scientific literature. They can be distilled down into a concentrated course of inoculation.

So why is the cutting edge of the latest research, which helps us master our minds, being ignored? Why are our leaders fixated on rules for the masses that may be misdirected and futile? Indeed, why might we be persuaded by our leaders at all?

When terrified, we tend to behave in a surprisingly predictable manner, which makes us easier to control. There are profound political implications. This psychology has been exploited by leaders and the manipulators in our lives from time immemorial. In other words, it may even be in the interest of the authorities for you to remain pliable, detained by dread.

This *Mental Vaccine for COVID-19* inoculates you from needless fear, clearing the 'psycho' path ahead for you. Instead of a freeze or faint reflex, crisis requires a fight plan with an effective response.

If Churchill had declared in the middle of the Blitz, as V rockets screamed down on London, 'Trust me when I say, love always wins...' Well, we'd all be speaking German now.

The Mental Vaccine for COVID-19 drags the issue into the universe of science, as well as pragmatic realism. This is the world I inhabit as a psychiatrist on a daily basis attempting to help people confronting very tough times in my clinic, not a recording studio.

Almost every single bit of psychological support you have been advised on through the popular media over the last year is not just wrong, it's badly off-beam. Often the exact opposite strategy might be more helpful. Making a list of all the things that worry you could help you retain them, not assist in dismissing them.

Our bodies are blessed with physical immune systems inherited from our ancestral past. We evolved white blood cells and antibodies over thousands of generations to survive the hazards of an infectious world. Vaccines mobilise our immune systems to protect us from new challenges. They would be useless if they didn't stimulate a natural defence that lies dormant within us.

Similarly, our minds retain intuitive immunity mechanisms, because our ancestors faced tough pressures before. But to benefit from inbuilt suppleness of the spirit, you need to know where your mind's natural defences lie, and how to activate them. You need to grasp how your mind works normally.

This, therefore, is a comprehensive guide to understanding and meeting the complex mental challenges of COVID-19, and growing individually stronger in the process, so after the pandemic is over, it will have left you more resilient, not weaker and more depleted, than if it had never happened.

I discuss in Part 1 how, no matter how terrible the circumstance, you can learn to control or regulate yourself. I explain how seeking an internal or physical place of safety is a priority, what that means, what it looks like, and how to create it, even if you can't physically go anywhere. I shall show how most comforting places people flee to, when trying to escape danger, end up being more hazardous than the peril they were attempting to escape from. Like crawling into a bottle. Or making a list.

When official instruction is all about isolating, it misunderstands that our need to affiliate is at its strongest when we are most distressed. Most official directives in this pandemic have attempted to cut directly across basic human emotional needs.

I confront headlong the question of suicidal thoughts and what to do about them, and whether crying works as a coping strategy. We learn, surprisingly, how it hinges on what kind of weeping, just as it depends, we discover later, on what sort of sense of humour helps.

Having covered how to wrestle with personal emotional upheaval, this first and important shot of the mental vaccine also comes in the form of the psychological implications of the new predicaments we have had to adapt to, like living under lockdown, washing your hands all the time, boredom, loneliness, fighting with those close to you.

People have been asked to make an extraordinary series of dramatic changes to almost every aspect of their lives without any assistance over the climactic consequences. For our mental health, the million-dollar question which has never been confronted by officialdom is: should we always do as we are told?

In Part 2, I demonstrate how to think more clearly about the strange and difficult world we now inhabit, and how to reason incisively and independently, and act more powerfully in that sphere. Insights into why a variety of authority figures seem to behave irrationally underscore the need for this additional vaccine booster shot. The mental vaccine involves imaginatively arriving at what works for you and those around you, as opposed to assuming the one-size-fits-all approach of the totalitarian state in which we have found ourselves.

The final booster you need is in Part 3, which is intended to lock in true long-term immunity from psychological harm, where I show how there has to be a major reassessment of the future. The psychological legacy will last decades. I will demonstrate how we need to protect generations to come, drawing on studies of our past collective traumas and pandemic experiences.

We are at a crucial crossroads in history. If we are not mentally vaccinated now, the trajectory of our lives, and those of our children, and even their children, could be knocked off course. Even if the pandemic comes under control soon, there are various possible side effects and we must be prepared to face them proactively. Crossing your fingers and praying for it all to be over soon is just not going to cut it. We need to change our life perspective.

The question on everyone's mind, but which no one seemed to dare ask, is did Meghan, in 'that' interview with Oprah Winfrey, betray whether she had herself found her own secret mental vaccine? Did that explain her survival following suicidal thoughts? Later in this guide, I explain the answer to that question, and its relevance to you.

I am sorry to say, 'Bah humbug,' Meghan and Harry, and you seem like nice people, but love doesn't always win. Indeed, it's one of the most self-destructive emotions. Shakespeare understood this. It's why, at the end of *Romeo and Juliet*, it's as if a plague has struck; the stage is littered with dead bodies. No matter how involving a story that was, it was not about an effective mental vaccine.

Fresh from the laboratory, after having been subjected to proper scientific trials involving thousands of participants, here is a much better one.

INTRODUCTION

A PLAGUE OF THE ABSURD

Is it pointless to pit yourself against the pandemic?

On 27 April 2020, Dr Lorna Breen, medical director of the emergency department at NewYork-Presbyterian Hospital in Manhattan, was in the newspaper headlines. The hospital had been inundated with COVID-19 cases.

She had just committed suicide.[1]

The 49-year-old's father, Dr Philip Breen, told the *New York Times*: 'She tried to do her job and it killed her.'[2] When they last spoke, his daughter had seemed 'detached', relating how COVID-19 patients were dying before they could even be removed from ambulances.

Lorna contracted COVID-19 in March, having only recently returned to work in April. Scheduled to slog through nine 12-hour shifts in a row, she stayed late every day. She was not just an eminent doctor; she ran marathons, loved skiing and danced salsa. Perhaps because of her work ethic, and knowing how much she was needed at her clinic, which was inundated with Coronavirus, she returned to her patients' bedsides too early.

Maybe all those leisure activities, so vital in distracting from the stress of such a demanding career, were also suddenly whipped away by pandemic precautions. Did this generate gaps in her usual coping strategies? The media may have been looking in the wrong place, purely blaming her workload for her demise. Others may be making the same error when it comes to grasping the true cause of anguish in an outbreak.

Resilience arises more from the effectiveness of the survival response you mount to trauma than from the intensity of the ordeal itself.

For example, there is an indispensable 'Four Tasks' coping strategy when it comes to dealing effectively with any loss, whether you've lost a job, access to leisure activities, a relationship or maybe even the life of a loved one. Perhaps the sense of being an effective clinician, which is now stolen from them, is a shock which physicians all over the world have been struggling with. This 'Four Task' action plan is not just an essential approach for anyone hoping to bear these misfortunes. It remains, in my daily clinical experience helping individuals besieged with multiple losses, the only viable technique.

The 'Four Tasks' of dealing with hurt are described in Chapter 3. These are surprisingly simple deeds anyone can undertake, but despite being terrifically pragmatic and effective, the framework remains astonishingly unfamiliar to many in the world of psychology, psychiatry and medicine. Dr Breen may have been unaware of this essential psychological survival toolkit.

What did she know that we don't? Are the rest of us simply in denial over the reality? Does feeling desolate become impossible to avoid when we face such overwhelming upheaval? Where to look for answers?

Albert Camus' novel *The Plague*, published in 1947, wrestles with this precise dilemma, though he thought the bug would cross over from a rat and not, allegedly, from a wet market in Wuhan. A doctor at the front line in the fight against a mysterious epidemic narrates this main coping resource, an essential survival guide that people are turning to today.[3]

The medic hero battling the plague in Camus' account, Dr Rieux, fights on against absurdly impossible odds. The virus wipes out half the population of a community forced into isolation. While the family physician becomes demoralised occasionally, he endures, remaining mentally intact by the end.[3]

But in reality, our hard-working specialist in Manhattan didn't. Why? Dr Lorna Breen's father, Dr Philip Breen, maintained his daughter did not have a history of mental illness, but that 'she was truly in the trenches of the front line'.[2]

If we hold up *The Plague* as a mirror to our real-life Coronavirus pandemic, are there any conclusions we can draw for our predicament? As the Nobel-winning author appeared to prophesy our current unhinged state, many people have turned to the book recently, to find out.[4]

Camus interprets the futile efforts by the fictional doctor in line with his own philosophy. For Camus life is absurd and pointless – this was why it was inevitable that anything Dr Rieux tried did not work.[4] For the existentialist Camus, survival relies on deeper acceptance of this reality. It's the incessant attempt to swing the odds your way, to fight the pandemics, which will kill you – as indeed it appeared, at first glance, to do with Dr Lorna Breen.

Researchers from the University of British Columbia[5] who investigated 6,854 American and Canadian adults, representing the general population, concluded that the 'psychological footprint' of COVID-19 is likely to be dramatically more substantial than the medical impact. The number of people emotionally affected by COVID-19 far exceeds the total number infected by the virus. The research found only 2 per cent of this large sample reported that they had been diagnosed with COVID-19, and only 6 per cent were personally acquainted with someone who had contracted COVID-19.

These figures are useful to keep the pandemic in perspective: while millions are infected around the planet, they remain a relatively small proportion of total global population. And yet 38 per cent experienced some degree of distress in this survey, while an additional 16 per cent were highly distressed and likely in need of mental health services. These are the disturbingly large numbers. These results mean you could multiply by 22 every time you see statistics on the number of viral cases to get a sense of what is really going on behind the scenes, mentally, in the population.

Yet because poor emotional health is not as evident as coughing up blood, the psychological impact of the contagion remains vastly underestimated, and under-reported.

The government and media easily overlook people with distressing mental health issues because, inhibited and avoidant, sufferers will not parade with placards on the streets. Death statistics are, on the other hand, measurable and demonstrable. The media like to report dramatic scenes, such as ambulances queueing with dying patients inside. The government knee-jerk is vast public borrowing and lockdowns thrown at this highly visible problem. In customary fashion, a long-term, coherent emotional health strategy is nowhere to be seen, just as we face an appalling and enduring psychiatric crisis.

Is there some psychological medicine that will heal that feeling of being unglued by our current catastrophe, something that will inoculate you against the terrible tension?

In official psychology and psychiatry no one is even attempting to disseminate the absolutely indispensable 'Four Task' model of coping with loss, for instance. This is alarming.

Japan has traditionally experienced very low rates of what are referred to as 'common mental disorders' – problems like anxiety and depression.[6] The prevalence of common mental disorders in the USA is approximately three times that of Japan. Also, Japan has, at the time of writing, relatively low rates of COVID-19 impact compared to other parts of the world, with around 7,595 deaths to date.[7]

Yet suicide rates in Japan have now climbed to their highest level in five years, with a total of 2,153 people killing themselves during October 2020, a monthly increase of more than 300: this in the world's third-largest economy. Until quite recently, the total number of suicides in Japan in just a couple of months was more than the total number of people who had died from COVID-19 since the beginning of the outbreak.[7] *The Japan Times* reported that the health ministry calculated 20,919 people died by suicide in 2020, compared with 3,460 deaths from coronavirus over the same period.[7]

The suicide statistics from Japan are relevant for the rest of the world, as this country gets such fatality numbers published faster than practically anywhere else, so these are ominous harbingers for what may be coming for the rest of the planet.

The Economist reported that as of 10 December 2020, 564 South Koreans had died of COVID-19, a widely quoted statistic suggesting to the outside world that this technologically advanced first-world country, through superior organisational skills, has had a 'good' pandemic. Yet roughly twice that number of South Koreans died from suicide every month between January and September.[8]

Meanwhile, under a headline in *The Daily Telegraph* dated 9 November 2020, 'Suicide calls for help triple in "mental health pandemic"', it is reported that the London Ambulance Service has seen a 68 per cent rise in suicides and attempted suicides, with crews now attending 37 cases a day, compared with 22 this time last year.[9]

Another excerpt from *The Plague*:

Figures drifted through his head and he thought that the thirty or so great plagues recorded in history had caused nearly a hundred million deaths. But what are a hundred million deaths? When one has fought a war, one hardly knows any more what a dead person is. And if a dead man has no significance unless one has seen him dead, a hundred million bodies spread through history are just a mist drifting through the imagination.

Jacqueline Rose says this of Camus's prophetic masterpiece in *The London Review of Books*:[10]

> One of the things *The Plague* conveys is that, at the very moment we appear to be taking the grimmest reality on board, we might also be deluding ourselves. Counting is at once a scientific endeavour and a form of magical thinking. It can be a way of bracing ourselves for and confronting an onslaught, and at the same time a doomed attempt at omnipotence, a system for classifying the horror and bundling it away. What exactly are we being told each time the latest figures are announced, rising consistently, dropping slightly, increasing again? Other than that we cannot get a grip on what is happening.

La Peste contributed to Albert Camus winning the Nobel Prize for Literature in 1957 as the second youngest recipient in the prize's history.[11] When the book was first published it was seen as an allegory, where the pestilence represented the Nazi occupation of France; not an unreasonable surmise, given Camus wrote it while living through that invasion.

Yet with the passage of years scholars have come to realise that *The Plague* was in fact all along about... a plague. I think the clue might have been in the title.[11]

In *The Plague* Camus seems to be arguing that surviving a pandemic means treating it like warfare. But in this war the enemy has infiltrated even into our homes, it's not clear who your true allies are, or even where the front line is; you're constantly in retreat, and you're taking hits from all directions. Additionally, even if you surrender, the flak keeps coming in.

In fact, at the heart of *The Plague* is this disturbingly uncomfortable message, that maybe those seeking solace in its pages perhaps should be warned against. Camus contends that fighting the plague is utterly pointless. All the public health interventions become merely increasingly absurd attempts to reassure the public that their rulers remain in control, when in fact the disease has taken charge. 'I can imagine what this plague must mean to you. "Yes," said Rieux. "An endless defeat."'

As we thumb the pages for answers in the novel, we may recognise our own resignation to the horrors of numbers dead, and the futility of trying to fight a deadly infection.

It is not just the pandemic which is absurd in Camus' view: absurdity in life is endemic and has spread everywhere. The ludicrousness at the heart of our existence includes our inevitable deaths (the way doctors talk about saving lives it looks like they are in denial of this inevitability), how we strive for meaning in an unfeeling uncaring universe (hence the rise of conspiracy theories to explain the virus, as the notion it was just a random chance event seems unbelievable), and how we hopelessly strive to find order among the chaos of our world (like pursuing public health rituals believing they protect us absolutely, when they don't).

There appears an underlying bitterness to the medicine which Camus wants to dispense. The pandemic appears not to represent a new desolation, but merely reveals, like an x-ray searching for a new disease, inherent weaknesses lurking in our psychological immune systems. These were always there, lying dormant before.

Camus describes at the beginning the townspeople, as yet unsuspecting of the cataclysm about to be unleashed on them: 'The truth is that everyone is bored, and devotes himself to developing habits.'[11]

Yet there is hope. Displaying supremely unselfish behaviour, Dr Bernard Rieux, the medical hero of the novel, *disregards personal risk to offer support to dying and highly infectious patients.* Yet precisely because this is so difficult to do, indeed almost impossible, is there any way we can sugar Camus' horrible-tasting pill?

Maybe the necessary coping skills can't just be suddenly wheeled into the room, like a ventilator assisting in an emergency. Survival may demand deeper personal changes; more fundamental life support.

In the novel, Jacques Cottard, a criminal before the pandemic struck the town, continues his selfish exploits, profiteering from the misery through smuggling, just as today some have exploited our current predicament. Camus foresaw the millions in government aid that would be siphoned off by fraud and scams.

It's not just the virus which has made a killing.

According to the Office for National Statistics, for the year ending June 2020, one of the three fraud-reporting bodies, UK Finance, declared a 44 per cent rise (to 107,327 fraud offences).[12] A US court dispute has revealed that a Spanish businessman who acted as an intermediary to secure protective coronavirus equipment for NHS staff was allegedly paid £21 million in UK taxpayer cash. The consultant may have been due a further $20 million in UK public funds owed to him from a Miami jeweller named as Michael Saiger.[13]

It is alleged Saiger requisitioned £200 million in UK taxpayer money to procure Chinese-made masks, gloves and gowns; a contract awarded directly to him rather than being tendered competitively, despite the fact his company had no PPE to sell. The Department of Health said in response to press inquiries over the scandal that proper checks are done for all contracts.[14]

It turns out the UK government was so unprepared for the pandemic that it had to rush to buy personal protective equipment in a panic and were probably royally ripped off by rogues who saw them coming. For example, they spent over £150 million on unusable masks, which according to the Labour Party[15] is roughly what it would have cost to extend free school meals over the Christmas and Easter holidays. The lining of the pockets of the crooks, though the incompetence of bumbling officials, could be seen as literally taking bread from poor children's mouths.

At least £2.5 billion of the UK's personal protective equipment originated from Chinese manufacturers,[16] with 80 contracts citing just one particular factory. Such over-reliance on a narrow supply chain meant prices increased all the time, sometimes even after contracts were signed. While we were being held hostage in our homes during lockdown, we were also being held hostage when it came to pricing of the protection equipment we needed to escape. We were kidnapped and held to ransom… several times over.

At least £175 million in taxpayer money has been spent on consultants. Deloitte has been paid £49 million for Covid projects (though there is no suggestion of wrongdoing).[17] Even clinics have now been accused of profiteering from the coronavirus crisis. German hospitals stand accused of keeping intensive care beds empty rather than treating patients, in order to secure extra funding. A government emergency scheme paid hospitals €560 (£500) a day for every ICU bed kept free and so available for coronavirus patients. The allegation is that the danger they could run out of intensive care beds was overstated by hospitals, who were merely playing the system.[18]

Which? consumer magazine has identified three hand sanitisers which contained too little alcohol to safely kill COVID-19, or other germs, leaving you thinking you had cleaned when in fact you remained unprotected, so endangering yourself and others.[19] All three products claimed to contain at least 70 per cent alcohol; one had just 10 per cent (Klenzy Hand Sanitising Gel) and the other two (Hansan Antibacterial Hand Sanitiser and Vaida Makeup Hand Sanitiser Gel) just over 30 per cent. According to the World Health Organisation, you need at least 60 per cent alcohol by volume in your hand sanitiser to kill bacteria and viruses. Some hand sanitisers found in the US contain methanol, an ingredient which is in fact toxic to humans.[19]

The pandemic has been exploited by sections of our society which lie in wait for new opportunities, a bit like a virus might lurk, ever ready to infect a new host.

UK police are now appealing for any information relating to a scam referred to as the 'nude game show'.[20] Men report being invited to a local hotel in Newham to take part in 'nude challenges' that are then filmed. Others have fallen victim to this scam in which someone claiming to be part of the entertainment industry appears to represent a fictitious reality TV game show with a £5,000 prize. In fact, the police now believe no such TV show exists, with the footage being retained merely for the sexual gratification of the scam artist.[20]

We are so preoccupied with the new parasite we fail to detect the veiled menace from the human vermin who remain ever present, lurking in our midst. The psychology of fear, which leads us to freeze like rabbits caught in the headlights, has been exploited mercilessly. We need to achieve better emotional control not just for our mental health, but for many other reasons; like protection from financial depredation.

'They're like East Anglia's Bonnie and Clyde,' complained Julie Penney of the Swann Inn, Suffolk, speaking to the press in November 2020 about a couple who took to dining at expensive restaurants in the area, every day of the week, but then bolting without paying the bill. Norfolk and Suffolk Police investigated a series of meals costing up to £197, and a hotel stay. The couple even asked to take home a bottle of wine from one bistro, promising to settle the total bill, and were never seen again.[21] As reported in *The Guardian*, one landlord placed a steering wheel lock on the couple's car in order to secure payment – only for the man to apparently fake a heart attack, so making an escape in an ambulance.[21] How low can you go? Using a much-needed ambulance in the middle of a pandemic to make your escape from a scam over not paying for a meal? Even characters in *The Plague* didn't become self-serving.

But the most deeply disturbing question, unresolved by Camus, is whether you need that kind of psychopathic mindset in order to survive an epidemic. Whatever you may think morally about all the scams listed above, they appear to be perpetrated by survivors.

After a nuclear holocaust is it inevitable that it's the rats and the cockroaches who emerge first from the rubble?

At the other end of the moral spectrum is another character in *The Plague*, Joseph Grand,[11] an infirm, elderly man with some 'goodness of heart'. His spontaneous response is to declare: 'One's got to help a neighbour, hasn't one?'

The problem is although Joseph Grand represents ordinary goodness in the average citizen, and he does try to help victims stricken by the disease, he has his own problems. It turns out he has been trying to write a novel. But he can't get past the first sentence, which he then spends the entire lockdown writing and re-writing endlessly.

Is this the kind of fruitless repetitive behaviour that has seemed to occupy much of our seclusion recently? Surely there has to be a better answer than that?

According to Emeritus Professor of Philosophy Stephen Wagner's reading of *The Plague*,[22] the true goal should be to rid ourselves of any possibility of passing on to others that emotional ailment which we carried. There was, harboured within all of us, something the pandemic has now revealed. We all suffered from a failure to learn how to live properly, when we had a life to inhabit, unimpeded by disease.

Albert Camus seems to have anticipated the modern mental health impact. Another excerpt from the story, after the plague has become endemic:

> Everyone Tarrou set eyes on had that vacant gaze and was visibly suffering from the complete break with all that life had meant to him. And since they could not be thinking of their death all the time, they thought of nothing.

Is there an alternative to thinking of nothing? Camus in *The Plague* declares:[11]

> The newspapers, needless to say, complied with the instructions given them: optimism at all costs. If one was to believe what one read in them, our populace was giving 'a fine example of

courage and composure'. But in a town thrown back upon itself, in which nothing could be kept secret, no one had illusions about the 'example' given by the public. To form a correct idea about the courage and composure talked about by our journalists you had only to visit one of the quarantine depots or isolation camps established by our authorities.

Has Boris Johnson been reading Camus? Here is what the Prime Minister said after he was notified by NHS Test and Trace on Sunday November 16 2020 that he must self-isolate, despite the fact he had caught COVID-19 only a few months earlier:

> It doesn't matter that we were all doing social distancing, it doesn't matter that I'm fit as a butcher's dog, feel great – so many people do in my circumstances, and it doesn't matter that I've had the disease and I'm bursting with antibodies. We've got to interrupt the spread of the disease and one of the ways we can do that now is by self-isolating for 14 days when contacted by Test and Trace.

Camus predicted our authorities would be spinning around, nothing they do really making any difference; merely needing to be seen to be doing something. Meanwhile, their policies may be destroying more lives than the virus, just as *The Plague* would have predicted.

On 17 October 2020, the press reported on how famous actress Anna-Jane Casey – for three decades a West End leading lady – had been reduced by the shut-down of the theatre industry to the much less glitzy role of delivery driver, earning £1 per parcel.[23] Casey's dazzling West End career included playing Velma Kelly in *Chicago*, Anita in *West Side Story* and Mrs Wilkinson in *Billy Elliot*. Anita Singh,[23] the Arts and Entertainment Editor of *The Daily Telegraph*, describes how Casey, one of the most positive people in show-business, appeared to have been especially shattered by a particular experience.

Singh relates that Casey had to deliver a parcel to a famous West End and Broadway songwriter whom she knew. All of a sudden, out of the blue, she is confronted by an instant which seems to clarify and define just how far she has fallen, particularly in her own eyes. Her reported reaction vividly captured just how discouraging this moment was:

I've known him for years and, oh, the shame of Anthony opening that door. He was really sweet about it and it shouldn't be a problem but, you know … as I drove away … I did sob … I thought, 'Two months ago he'd have been asking me to go and do a demo for him for a new musical, and now I'm offering him a Lakeland parcel.'

Yet Anna-Jane Casey wanted her story of humiliation reported to draw attention to the need to open theatres again and save her industry. She grieves that she has been miscast as a delivery driver; but she deserves a standing ovation for this, the heroic performance of a lifetime. Another prescient passage from *The Plague*:

> … there's no question of heroism in all this. It's a matter of common decency. That's an idea which may make some people smile, but the only means of fighting a plague is common decency.

But what to do when stockpiles of common decency run low? (See Chapter 9 on the shocking rise of revenge porn during the pandemic and Chapter 13 on the psychology of trolling Captain Sir Tom Moore.)

There are, in fact, some very basic simple psychological turns of mind which are essential to coping with COVID-19; yet these have been ignored by the media, who, in concert with officialdom, have disseminated ineffective or even destructive mental health advice.

The family of Dr Lorna Breen have since responded to their tragedy by establishing the Lorna Breen Heroes' Fund, providing mental health support to healthcare professionals. Corey Feist, Lorna's brother-in-law, explained: 'She cared so deeply about her colleagues … We feel like this work is spreading her … It's the hardest thing I've ever done in my life. And it's the most rewarding.'[24]

Whether they were aware of it or not, this act is one of the final 'Four Tasks' of coping effectively with loss.

In this guide, I hope to show healing mentally during the pandemic requires living our whole life in a better way. The pandemic is a deep challenge to us to re-think what we thought daily existence was all about, in a fundamental sense. Accepting the task, adapting and changing completely, means survival. Evidenced methods for doing precisely this are the 'mental vaccine' options in the chapters ahead.

Camus' fiction is a despairing, disturbing allegory. Unnerved, we see our collective reflection in his imagined dystopia which turned out to be all too real.

But it does tell us something useful.

In the novel the fictitious population are complicit with life's pointlessness, but we, thankfully, do not have to be – and there lies huge opportunity. This is the positive message that I, and other survivalists, read into it – fortitude depends on profound personal transformation.

If you take away the right message, the pandemic can leave you mentally stronger, emotionally fitter, just as a vaccine stimulates your immune system.

It's very unusual to be hit by such a stressful event which bombards us from all sides, with losses at many levels: for example, loss of job or income, loss of social contact, loss of the ability to go outside and perform hobbies or interests or sports which entertained or occupied you, loss of connection with family members, loss of certainty over your future, or even just the loss of the ability to visit the cinema or to do the shopping. These losses and stresses are liable to have a profound impact on the population, with psychiatrists predicting elevated rates of psychiatric illness and even suicide as a consequence; and these effects have been shown by recent research to endure even years after a quarantine has ended.

The official advice on how to look after yourself at this difficult time includes, first and foremost, to stay at home when instructed to; but also to find things to do which absorb, engage and distract you, structuring your day to reduce boredom, remaining as physically active and fit as possible, limiting exposure to alarming media messages, as well as maintaining your social networks via digital technology. In fact, the latest advice is to be perhaps even more sociable via social media than usual, to tackle boredom and loneliness.

This demonstrates why maintaining well-being is such a precarious business; a dramatic change in circumstance can produce a profound turnaround in the standard counsel on how to retain mental health. Just a few months ago social media was seen as profoundly mentally endangering to us all, and in particular to young people. Given that the evidence is that the young are the most vulnerable to the long-term negative mental health effects of quarantine, it now seems that their mobile phone has suddenly been transformed into a life-line, as opposed to a danger.

The flip-flopping over recommendations is really about keeping going until the pandemic or the lockdown is over. What if there was a better approach, which was so effective you could keep doing it indefinitely if you really had to, not just crossing your fingers waiting for the horror to end?

Just in case you consider that a fanciful idea, remember that British journalist John McCarthy was kept hostage for five years in Lebanon from 1986 to 1991 and survived. For much of that time he was chained to a wall and blindfolded, while being kept in small pits for extended periods. What are the lessons from survivors of such an ordeal?

Stephen Wagner,[22] the Professor of Philosophy we encountered earlier, argues that what Albert Camus was really endeavouring to indicate is that what matters now, in the middle of a virulent scourge, is not striving to live the *best* life. This is just one of the fundamental errors behind all the authorised enlightenment. Instead, we should be striving for the *most* life.

What does that mean?

Oliver Sacks,[25] the famous neurologist, wrote in a short book of collected essays entitled *Gratitude*, as he contemplated his own death following a diagnosis of terminal cancer: 'Above all, I have been a sentient being, a thinking animal, on this beautiful planet, and that in itself has been an enormous privilege and adventure.'

Stephen Wagner may also be referring to a philosophy of resilience as expressed in the book *Meditations*[26] by the Roman emperor Marcus Aurelius (AD 121–180). Frequently writing huddled in his tent on battlefields before leading his army into potential destruction, the adherent of stoicism reflects:

> Our actions may be impeded ... but there can be no impeding our intentions or dispositions. Because we can accommodate and adapt. The mind adapts and converts to its own purposes the obstacle to our acting... The impediment to action advances action. What stands in the way becomes the way.

Stoicism is an ancient doctrine of which modern Cognitive Behavioral Therapy is basically a somewhat clunky, and watered down, re-hash.

In planning for the next war, the UK Committee of Imperial Defence[27] as far back as 1924 acknowledged stoicism as lying at the heart of mental resilience against the stress of aerial bombardment. Back in the 1920s, there seems to have been more intelligent reflection by officialdom upon public psychology than there was during the 2020s.

Everyone is complaining that watching grim statistics and incessant footage of desperate Intensive Care Units nightly on the TV news is merely compounding our despair. They want to turn away and switch off. Camus, ever the tough guy, claimed that this is the first mistake. Instead, he said, we must face the suffering and yet survive.[28] He set out what survival should look like but omitted to explain how to perform the necessary trick: gaining the strength to face the pandemic without being overwhelmed.

I attempt to start where *The Plague* finished.

Switching away from the horror of TV news, we need to find a better channel. But what does the new channel look like? The first step is grasping that survival is a decision. Decide to survive. But decide to survive and retain virtue as well. Indeed, survive through enhanced virtue.

The new channel does not resemble the scatter-gun, incoherent and shallow mental health advice of this pandemic. Channel-surfing is all the flip-flopping advice in our modern media amounts to. Instead, we need a more coherent practical philosophy that helps us surf whatever new tsunami is bearing down on us, shows us how to psychologically inoculate yourself against the virulence.

The joke doing the rounds is that, rather like buses, you wait months for a vaccine, and then three come along at the same time. At the time of writing there are so many different vaccines being rolled out across the world it's difficult to keep count.

Are we nevertheless in peril of still not learning the correct lesson?

That so many vaccines could be generated so quickly was partly because the virus was structured in a particular way, allowing older as well as relatively newer technology (mRNA vaccines), which stimulated our bodies to mount an effective immunising response. If the vaccines eventually prove as effective as the early data suggests, then it's because we got incredibly lucky on several fronts at once. We were blessed with a miracle roulette spin where the structure of COVID-19 and the availability and compatibility of bio-technology happened to coincide.

The next virus or mutation to come along may not be so magnanimous.

The correct lesson to learn is the precise opposite of what everyone has over-optimistically concluded – that science has triumphed and the virus is vanquished. What would happen if a mutation in this bug, or another germ, came along which was not quite so amenable to assisting the scientists? What scale of disaster across the planet would then ensue? This virus was just clearing its throat.

Perhaps we should heed Albert Camus' very last ominous prediction in the closing passages of *The Plague*:

> [That] the plague ... never dies or disappears for good; that it can lie dormant for years ... that it bides its time ... and that perhaps the day would come when, for the bane and the enlightening of men, it would rouse up its rats again and send them forth to die in a happy city.

PART 1

HOW TO COPE WITH CORONA

I

WHY WORRY IS MORE CONTAGIOUS THAN ANY VIRUS

Can antelope reveal how to outrun a lion and be more relaxed?

Animals do not worry.

In that simple, perhaps controversial, statement lies the secret to coping with COVID-19. The 'animals do not worry' line comes from a revolutionary paper[1] recently published in the *Journal of Anxiety Disorders* that suggests mental health experts have been barking up the wrong tree when it comes to advising the public on grappling with the germ.

Neuroscience's thinking about why we get anxious has now been turned on its head.

Animals do experience stress: and this occurs, just as in humans, when they find themselves confronting danger. The fear or anxiety response, genetically built into our bodies, is evolutionarily ancient. Even though it renders us upset, it's designed to ensure we remain vigilant for threat, and so stay safe and therefore alive. Panic meant we fled, fast, when a lion started bounding towards us across the African savannah, as we crossed its path as ancient cavemen, dragging our knuckles along the ground.

Grazing antelope may look content, but they also devote time to what zoologists refer to as 'vigilance' behaviour, which means looking up while they are chewing to check for predators, like lions or cheetahs.[2] They seem relaxed as they graze[3] in a way we wouldn't be if we had to keep checking the room during supper to ensure we were not about to be diced and served. If this was the case, imagine the difference in atmosphere at the Manoir aux Quat'Saisons...

This issue of why animals don't get stressed in the same way we do, despite the fact they appear to us to live in a more unpredictable and dangerous world, has preoccupied many neuroscientists, as explored in the recent bestselling book *Why Zebras Don't Get Ulcers* by Robert Sapolsky.[4] A Professor of Locomotor Biomechanics at the Royal Veterinary College in London, Dr Alan Wilson's research[3] has established that both cheetahs and lions have about 20 per cent more powerful muscles and 37 per cent greater acceleration capacity than their prey, like zebra and impala. Yet these formidable felines are successful in about only about a third of hunts.

Professor Wilson's team, collaborating with one at the University of Botswana, used specially designed radio collars to track animals' speeds during their chases. They found that while predators are significantly faster and more powerful than their prey, at lower velocities they're unable to match zebra and impala for manoeuvrability, allowing their prey an emergency exit. Professor Wilson explained:[3]

> In the final stages of a hunt, it isn't about high speed ... if the prey tries to run away at speed, it is a very bad move because the predator is faster and can accelerate more quickly, so that plays into the predator's hands ... the optimum tactics of the prey is to run relatively slowly and turn very sharply at the last moment ... prey ... define the chase ... it decides when to turn, how fast to run. It's always one stride ahead of the predator.

Now maybe we know why zebras don't get ulcers.

But wildlife doesn't stalk us in modern life, instead we confront social threat: a bullying boss; unemployment; social isolation or marital discord; a diffuse contagion that destroys our lives.

Yet all these predicaments still trigger the ancient 'fight or flight' escape response to physical peril. However, escape from a bullying boss, or a bug, is no longer as simple as bolting (though we wish it were).

Now a radically new theory[1] about the fundamental nature of stress, pioneered by psychologists Jos Brosschot and Bart Verkuil from Leiden University in the Netherlands and Julian Thayer from the University of California at Irvine, argues we have all been looking in the wrong place for mental health. According to these psychologists, the essential question is not why we get anxious when the world becomes dangerous; instead, the fundamental dilemma is *recognising what safety looks like*. For antelope, for example, there is security in extreme cornering.

This revolutionary new way of thinking is particularly relevant to the mental health aspects of coping with COVID-19.

The invisible virus has turned many everyday aspects of life into new dangers, such as commonplace physical contact and normal socialising. Ordinary activities such as going to school or commuting to work have now apparently become hazardous. Even if you try to avoid threats by remaining at home, new risks emerge in the form of social isolation, losing your job, and the impact of an obliterated economy.

Experiments have established that the new coronavirus can endure in the air for three hours and can survive for up to four hours on copper, twenty-four hours on cardboard and two to three days on plastic and stainless steel.[5] Another study[6] has also established that it can journey 5 metres through the air. Infectious particles were isolated up to 4.8 metres from patients being treated at the University of Florida Health Shands Hospital. This is significantly further than the advised 2-metre social distancing rule.

Meanwhile, another investigation,[7] published in the *Journal of Korean Medical Science*, tracking airflow in a restaurant from air conditioning, found virally infected droplet transmission over more than 21 feet. One visitor overlapped with an infected diner for only five minutes, yet caught COVID-19.

If you thought a viral infection meant you became immunised, and so at long last were finally safe from catching it again, beware. According to one report,[8] the first death from COVID-19 reinfection has happened in the Netherlands, and a 25-year-old man in Nevada has caught the virus twice.

Nowhere seems safe, triggering the ancient threat-detecting anxiety system within our brains, leading to chronic stress and therefore mental breakdown.

Medical experts keep broadcasting frightening statistics on TV designed to scare us into submission. But the subtext is your government now finds your very existence a problem: you represent a way of spreading the virus as well as a black hole of need and vulnerability. You have become the enemy. You can run but you cannot hide. No one explains what is harmless; but they cannot stop highlighting what is dangerous. A better approach would have been to view the public as a solution rather than a problem.

Brosschot, Verkuil and Thayer[1] argue we have developed a generalized perception of 'unsafety' and maybe, following their thesis, our leaders have as well.

A traumatic experience is transformed by the mind into worry that it's going to happen again, so we become vigilant for danger no matter where we are. This means no situation can be really benign, as the mind has transformed everywhere into locations of potential menace.

If your boss has begun bullying you at work, then his or her mere presence signals danger, so you become stressed, even when the boss is not tormenting you but just saying hello. Your brain starts viewing the entire office as a place of danger, generalising to commuting (so the train makes you sick to your stomach); finally, just thinking about anything which is linked to your job becomes a trigger for worry. Eventually, everything becomes an indicator you are not in a place of safety, no matter where you are.

The three pioneering authors label their new theory 'Generalized Unsafety Theory of Stress', or GUTS,[1] suggesting that not being able to switch off the worry response is the basic issue because stress spills over into objectively safe places and times.

This essential difference between animals and us – they get anxious, but they don't worry – holds the secret to mental health. Rumination transforms relatively safe situations into unsafe predicaments. Worry is the most common aversive mental experience, and yet most therapy does not reveal the essential life skill of how to deal with worry effectively.

This firstly requires us to grasp the technical definition of worry.

Before we discuss how to handle worry more healthily, I challenge my patients in our clinic by asking them to define precisely what a worry is. Labelling more clearly exactly what is going on in our minds is a vital first phase to the improved management of internal mental phenomena. It is simply amazing how often this is side-stepped in most therapy. No patient I have ever asked to define what worry is has been able to do it properly (and most doctors can't either). Even after years of therapy elsewhere, when the patient has come for a second opinion, it is astonishing how blankly they look back when I ask them to explain what the mental phenomenon of a worry is.

This attempt dispassionately to label the different phenomena that are streaming through your consciousness is absolutely indispensable in achieving better emotional control and superior mental health. In attempting this we achieve several objectives, including a certain distance from our own inner experience, which immediately gives us more power over ourselves.

We are learning to think about our thinking. This is referred to as 'meta-cognition' in the field. Any time you go to see a therapist or doctor and they don't appear to be embarking on this enterprise at the beginning of any psychological treatment, then make your excuses and leave.

Many people struggle to define worry, not just patients in my clinics. Here comes the precise definition. This is an essential component in the COVID-19 Mental Vaccine. The rigorous definition of worry is: 'a negative anticipation of the future'.

Effectively handling apprehension requires us firstly to question whether our adverse expectation is realistic. Then, is there anything we can do, practically, in terms of active problem-solving, to stop the undesirable prediction coming true? If we are worrying about a future exam, then might revising become the antidote to worry?

Once we have done all the problem-solving (swotting) we can, we need then to retreat to a place of safety. That is to grasp that worrying no longer serves any positive function, and will merely upset us.

Yet that favourite refuge for most students – watching TV or visiting social media instead of studying – means they are pursuing the opposite strategy. A place of seeming shelter from the storm is in fact treacherous. The more comforted they are by the distraction of TV, as learning opportunities slip by, the more they are sliding to an ever more perilous cliff-edge than they realise.

The correct location for safety from the danger of the exam is in fact the study or desk, where they should be cramming. But instead, these settings – the desk, the study, the library – all represent danger and so are avoided. The hazard they all represent is being reminded of your ignorance, so you avoid those places as they seem perilous, and beat a retreat instead to the TV room, which just appears reassuringly safe. But appearances are misleading as exams loom.

A massive part of the self-destructiveness at the heart of the human condition is the pervasive tendency to seek safety in hideaways that then turn out to be much more lethal compared to whatever you were running from in the first place. Antelope don't seem to make that mistake. This would be like running from a lion towards a cheetah.

So why does it feel like we spend all day swerving between predators?

There are a group of people referred to by psychologists as 'chronic worriers', and they tend to spend much more time obsessing than the rest of us. Intriguingly, although they are often more prone to depression and anxiety because of excessive rumination, they also tend to end up much more successful than the average non-worrier. This is because – whisper it, as the therapy mafia won't want this disseminated – a certain amount of worry is in fact beneficial. It leads to anticipation of future difficulties lurking on the road up ahead, and therefore invites better planning to prevent them transforming into calamities.

It is vital to grasp that the essential difference between healthy and unhealthy worry has to do with another fundamental concept: that of one's orientation to time. Chronic worriers are forever living in the future, but there are two other temporal orientations to think about, namely the present and the past.

The pandemic requires us to be able to shift between time orientations in a new way.

Psychologists believe that fundamentally there are two kinds of people in the world: those who divide everybody into two kinds of people, and those who don't. Apologies, that was a terrible and very old joke. Apparently, it first appeared in a spoof review by humorist Robert Benchley in *Vanity Fair* magazine in February 1920. The quote comes from an extremely literary review of the New York City Telephone Directory. Benchley was apparently dissatisfied with the 'plot', declaring, 'It lacks coherence.' He went on to complain, 'We are herein presented to some five hundred thousand characters ... It is hard to tell which one is the most lovable.' I shall discuss sense of humour as an essential coping mechanism later in Chapter 6.

In the meantime, it is true that psychologists believe that you can divide people into three basic groups in terms of their time-orientation: you're either past-oriented, present-oriented or future-oriented.

Past-oriented people are very influenced by past events. They failed an exam ten years ago, and have decided they're never going to face another test again in their lives. They remain convinced they're never going to pass. In a lockdown depriving you of all the fun things you used to enjoy, being past-oriented, or nostalgic for the past, is liable to end up rendering you depressed. Yet if you switch to being future-oriented, it is also impossible to plan for what may be coming, as the horizon remains so uncertain.

Present-oriented people live for the moment. They really enjoy life, but because they're living for the instant, they blithely ignore the future consequences of present behaviour. To an extent, the pandemic requires us when coping with stress to be more 'in the present', and less in the future or in the past.

Future-oriented people, in contrast, worry a lot. They fret over the future. They're dwelling on the impending. They've got pensions, they've got insurance… They're concerned about the consequences of present behaviour, and the fact that they ruminate is no accident. They tend to be much more aware than the rest of us about the eventual consequences. They are busy revising for exams and don't do anything to encourage lung cancer.

If the technical definition of a worry is a negative anticipation of the future, it's intriguing to note that successful, motivated people tend to be very future-oriented. While they tend to fear excessively, negatively anticipating things and so acting to prevent bad things happening later, this often makes them supremely functional.

An exam may be a year away, but future-oriented chronic worriers feel destiny is very close, so they're working feverishly for the test now, anticipating possible negative events on the horizon – like failing the assessment – so they're acting immediately to try and prevent it, by revising.

Given that very motivated people are more future-oriented, does anyone want to have a guess at what's the best time-orientation for your overall mental health and wellbeing?

A lot of people are waving their hands in the air, shouting out, 'Present!' Well, it's great to be present-oriented because you have more fun and you enjoy life more than future-oriented people, but the problem with being present-oriented is this: if there is a massive negative consequence for some behaviour, it is very wise to be future-oriented at that moment.

This partly explains the strain of the pandemic – the need to switch to future orientation and consider preventing catching the bug whenever you are asked to take a precaution over what was before an everyday part of life.

Now, you're all going to go away and buy one of my previous books,[9] *The Motivated Mind*, and as a result, you will all have your own private aircraft at some point in the near future! Imagine you go out in the winter to have a flight in your private jet, and it's a cold winter's morning, and you get into the warm, snug cockpit, and then you suddenly remember the instructor reminding you that on a cold winter's morning you must check the wings of the aircraft have been properly de-iced: if you don't, that could cause a tail-spin at 30,000 feet and you might plummet to your death.

But as you enjoy the warm, snug cockpit, you say to yourself, oh, I don't want to go out into the cold winter morning and de-ice the wings. Here we have a moment where it's absolutely crucial that you are not too present-oriented and instead start being a little bit future-oriented and get out there and check the aircraft.

The correct answer in terms of overall wellbeing is the ability to shift between past, present and future depending on the situation in which you find yourself. The problem with being future-oriented incessantly is you never enjoy life. The extremely important idea here is that of transitioning fluidly from one state to the other depending on what is required of you by your environment – but also what will best attain your goal.

For example, suppose you are on a group call with a bunch of friends who begin reminiscing about all that tennis you played together before the lockdown. This nostalgic looking back is required of you in order to stay in the conversation, and continue to bond with your fellow tennis players. This means you have to shift for a time, to indulge in being past-oriented. However, as you realise this is just going to bring everyone down in the longer term, as they dwell on what they are missing, you could take control and suddenly shift to being future-oriented and suggest you all plan a tennis holiday abroad for when the lockdown is over.

After that you could consider transitioning to being present-oriented and suggesting an online computer game version of tennis you could all play to replace the physical doubles you are all missing. Or you could suggest the group watch an old famous tennis match on the internet.

Notice how this coping strategy requires you to become more consciously aware of past, present and future, and also to be become active in making the shift as necessary; and being more aware of your goals, as well as reconciling these with the demands of your environment.

In worry, the central question we all need to ask ourselves to achieve mental survival in a pandemic is this: what does *true safety* look like? In a mental sense is it the past, present or future?

The answer will differ from person to person, but it is the inability to identify safety, and learning to inhabit it, which explains chronic stress. Safety could be a location, perhaps a lifeboat after the *Titanic* went down, or under the duvet as a refuge from a brutal world, or it can be a mental place: meditation, or watching a distracting movie, or being absorbed by a hobby or sport.

Recent reviews of the scientific evidence for the efficacy of meditation and other similar now trendy 'mindfulness' therapies, have discovered that these are not quite the refuge they are cracked up to be. They are another example of a supposedly 'safe' refuge which turns out to be promising more sanctuary than is actually delivered.

One of the most recent comprehensive reviews of research on the benefits of meditation concludes that rigorous clinical trials find only 'small to moderate reductions of multiple negative dimensions of psychological stress'.

Mantra-based meditation programs such as Transcendental Meditation did not significantly improve any of the outcomes examined. Transcendental Meditation, unlike other meditation techniques, emphasises the use of a mantra in such a way that it 'transcends one to an effortless state where focused attention is absent'. An analysis entitled 'Meditation Programs for Psychological Stress and Well-being: A Systematic Review and Meta-analysis'[10] was published in the prestigious *Journal of the American Medical Association – Internal Medicine*. It was conducted because many now use meditation to treat stress-related conditions and promote general health.

Madhav Goyal, Jennifer Haythornthwaite and a team from Johns Hopkins University and Medical School in the USA reviewed forty-seven separate studies with 3,515 participants.[10] Their analysis found that 'Mindfulness' meditation programs showed moderate evidence of improved anxiety, depression, and pain, but low evidence of improved stress and mental health-related quality of life. They found no evidence that TM improved any outcomes.

These relatively small effects of 'Mindfulness' meditation are comparable with what would be expected from the use of an antidepressant, but without the associated toxicities. The review did conclude that meditation does appear free of possible harms or harmful side-effects compared with other treatments.

'Mindfulness' meditation derives from aspects of Buddhism, and involves learning to become aware of thoughts and internal states but not be affected emotionally by them – so-called non-judgemental awareness. Mindfulness has been described as the next new wave in psychological treatment – following on from CBT or Cognitive Behavioural Therapy.

This review found there was little to no evidence of any significant effect of any kind of meditation on positive mood, attention, substance use, eating habits, sleep or weight. There was no evidence that meditation programs were better than any active treatment (i.e. drugs, exercise and other behavioural therapies). Behavioural treatments tend to emphasise performing an action – such as confronting what is making you anxious – while 'Mindfulness' meditation appears to encourage facing challenges, but from a different mental angle – you aren't judging it, you are not reacting to it.

'Mindfulness' meditation techniques did appear most effective in dealing with a particular kind of pain referred to as 'visceral', in other words pain coming from organs such as the stomach or bowels, but it was less effective with pain from muscles and bones. This suggests that perhaps certain techniques of meditation may be useful in particular conditions, but they are not panaceas.

Meditation is a skill or state learned and practised over time, increasing awareness and gaining insight and understanding into the various subtleties of existence. Training the mind in awareness, in non-judgmental states, or in the ability to become completely free of thoughts or other activity are 'daunting accomplishments'. The authors of the study recommend longer-term trials with an emphasis on greater amounts of mental training. They also point out that the interest in meditation that has grown during the past thirty years in Western cultures derives from Eastern traditions emphasising lifelong growth. The West may have fundamentally misunderstood the basic point of meditation, and trying to do short-term trials just compounds the misunderstanding. Madhav Goyal, Jennifer Haythornthwaite and the team from Johns Hopkins University conclude from their review that meditation programs could help reduce anxiety, depression and pain, but only in some people.

On the other hand, Kristin Barker[11] of the University of New Mexico has published a critique of 'Mindfulness' meditation, pointing out several inherent contradictions in the practice. Her paper 'Mindfulness meditation: Do-it-yourself medicalization of every moment' points out that 'Mindfulness' meditation contends one is healed through accepting things as they are, even (or especially) in the presence of illness; yet many of the books and recordings advocating the technique boast descriptions of seemingly phenomenal cures through mindfulness. Published in the academic journal *Social Science & Medicine*, the critique points out a host of contradictory phrases arising from 'Mindfulness': 'One needs to try less and be more', intentionally cultivating the attitude of non-striving, and, one must engage in 'doing nothing, on a regular basis, on a systematic basis, in a disciplined way'.

But why meditate when you could just learn to rest properly? This is precisely the title of an idea[12] I published in the academic journal *Archives of Internal Medicine*. Does the need for all these 'techniques' with trendy names merely obscure the basic fact we just need to learn how to relax properly and deeply? Have we forgotten that skill in our frenetic world?

Therapists have gone into business to monetise training programs and books which are just basically about … how to take a proper breather. A billion-dollar business has been created flogging us apps, books, courses, CDs, and T-shirts but is in fact just selling back to us something our ancestors and grandparents never dreamed we would need to purchase. This is an industry devoted to disguising the massive health benefits of something you could learn to do at no cost. It is precisely because it's free that there is no marketing push behind it, and as a result it has been neglected.

This is the power of unwinding. Proper rest.

In the academic journal reference above, I was responding to a study which reported that the use of Transcendental Meditation for sixteen weeks in patients with heart disease improved blood pressure and other health indices. This was compared with a control group receiving health education.

Yet a wide variety of different meditation and relaxation techniques, marketed under contrasting brand names, converge on achieving slower breathing, generalised muscular relaxation and focused attention. You don't necessarily need to pay money, nor formally learn some complex technique, to be able to become better at these things. In fact, many of the widespread physiological effects of meditation are indistinguishable from simple 'resting' according to recent investigations.[13] Indeed, it remains an open question whether it is possible to distinguish the mental and physical states achieved between winding down deeply and meditation.[13] It is therefore entirely possible that many of the supposed health benefits attributed to meditation and mindfulness techniques could have just as likely been achieved by merely advising people to properly relax in a focused manner for the equivalent amount of time. Scientific investigations of mindfulness and meditation need to incorporate a resting comparison group, but they often don't, disguising the fact that any benefits from meditation or 'Mindfulness' could be explained from simple calming down.

This is a particularly important consideration given how time-consuming the Transcendental Meditation arm of the study I was responding to became. It involved two introductory lectures (1.5 hours each), personal interview (usually 10–15 minutes), personal instruction (1–1.5 hours), three group meetings (1.5 hours each), and follow-up and maintenance meetings (1.5 hours) twice per week for the first four weeks and weekly thereafter. Advising people to take up meditation or mindfulness may not be realistic, given this time commitment and the motivation required. However, the simple advice to rest properly might be more likely to be followed, is less expensive, has few adverse effects, and could be just as effective.

Maybe the power of jargon terms and a CD you have to buy is that it seems like the doctor has prescribed something more concrete, and therefore you are more likely to follow through, as opposed to if you were just dismissed from the consultation with the injunction to 'rest properly'. Yet there is a deep wisdom in that advice.

One client I had, and I have their permission to relate this anecdote, was extremely successful, but very driven, competitive and as a result somewhat 'highly strung'. Following a high-stress heart attack, they were referred to me to get them to calm down. They were so 'hyper' that it was clear that just suggesting they learn to deeply relax was not going to get us anywhere. In that case I prescribed a meditation course, because I knew what was inevitably going to unfold.

Sure enough, the group element of attending classes was manna to his competitive psyche. He got into what can only be described as 'competitive meditating'. He would obsessively check with everyone afterwards just how submerged a state they had achieved. He wanted to ensure his trance was the most profound. Like many, I think he had developed a mental block over what it is to genuinely let go and achieve serenity.

Resting – in case you busy people have forgotten what this means – involves paying deep attention to the goal of relaxing. It requires breathing more slowly but in a measured and controlled manner, relaxing the body physically, clearing the mind of thought, and avoiding distractions – all of which, of course, duplicates meditation instructions and strategies. It's just that the instructors use more fancy jargon terms, allowing them to charge high fees.

I am, however, advocating that you take resting seriously and research on the internet the various slow-breathing methods that exist. Breathing should be broken down into inhalation, holding and exhalation, and must be done to specific counts so that each breath is precisely measured to be the same. Regularised deliberate breaths are an ancient practice and remain at the heart of learning to calm down. Once you have got the breathing sorted – usually the required respiration rate is much, much, slower than you ever imagined possible – you need progressively to relax your muscles. There are several internet resources on this. Stick to ones published by people who have done academic work in the area. Finally, use your mind to vividly imagine a deeply relaxing scene with you in the middle of the experience.

You should learn to put your feet up, and reserve some of the day to project chill. But the key difference is, you need to be much more focused on the goal, which is to achieve a state of complete inner calm and the removal of physical tension. Paradoxically, you also need to devote a part of each twenty-four-hour period to the exact opposite of calm. It is because you are going out of your way to create a scheduled period of active panic, this will, counter-intuitively, also then generate a relative oasis of calm for the rest of your waking hours.

One powerful way to create a place of safety during the day if you are a chronic worrier is to deploy a technique referred to as 'worry timetable'. What this means is that you allocate a particular time of the day where you schedule your misgivings. It might be, say, between 5 p.m. and 5.30 p.m. each day. If worries occur to you at another time, you agree to park them, and only give your mind over to worrying about them at a particular set time. Scheduling apprehension is a powerful way of creating mental space free of brooding and therefore a place of safety. This is a much more helpful technique as simply not agonising is usually just not possible, whereas postponing worry is often viable.

Your brain will allow you to postpone the worry as opposed to accepting simply not worrying, though this will take a little practice at first to get the hang of it. But once you have your regular worry timetable schedule of when you are allowed to worry, you will be surprised at how rapidly and how easily your mind falls into step with postponing worry to a specific, regular part of the day.

Then having postponed it, bringing it back to mind consciously means that much of the emotionally toxic element to the worry will have been lost, and they will be considerably easier to endure, and also more receptive to being handled in a much healthier manner.

Once you have recalled your worry during worry timetable you should then say to yourself, what practical problem-solving can I do now to prevent my feared anticipation of the future actually occurring? If there is nothing pragmatic you can do, like revising for an exam, it makes no sense to continue with that worry, so park it until the next worry timetable schedule comes around. After a while, believe it or not, using the powerful technique of a worry timetable means that you end up with empty time when you were meant to be worrying.

You should not use the worry timetable for worries over things that crop up during the day which require a pragmatic response immediately. For those issues, act straight away. Reserve worry timetable for those ruminations that come and sit around in your head and cannot be dismissed easily, yet for which there is no immediate action that makes obvious sense.

We can even further unpick the workings of worry and get close to what *true safety* might be, for us.

A study entitled 'Some key differences between a happy life and a meaningful life'[14] examined happiness levels in a large sample and found that this issue of how much you lived in the past, present or future was absolutely crucial in determining how happy you were. The authors of the study[14] contend that happiness is about the present; whereas what they refer to as the meaningful life is about linking events across time, thus integrating past, present and future.

Meaning in life is about having longer-term goals. For example, those pursuing a meaningful life want to build something that lasts over time and so they may have families; whilst those pursuing the merely happy life should avoid relatives – and also clichés – like the plague. One decisive mental impact of the pandemic has been to make us much more aware and worried about the future than before.

The investigation[14] explains that happiness is mostly in the moment, and therefore largely independent of other moments. The more time people reported having devoted to thinking about the past and future, the more meaningful their lives were, but the less joyful. In contrast, the more time people reported thinking about the present, the happier they were.

In a pandemic we need to be able to make the present a place of safety, while the future becomes a much more precarious and dangerous place to dwell on.

We must find and inhabit places of mental or physical safety: know where they are, and go to them, once we can do no more problem-solving. We also have to be able to work out new ways of finding meaning if our previous pursuits are now blocked by the pandemic.

For survival reasons the stress response is always there, lurking in the background, on the verge of being activated, only being properly switched off when safety is clearly apparent. As long as there is no clear proof of safety, insecurity remains, and the default stress response remains 'on'.

What has to be learnt as we grow and develop is what safety looks like.

Ever-evolving uncertainty about the future, given a mutating virus, swings in government policy and public health advice, means that the goalposts keep shifting over what is, or what is not, alarming. Intolerance of uncertainty underpins panic during this crisis.

As reported widely in the press,[15] on 28 November 2020, a care home owner, Vernon Hough, killed himself due to the 'incredible emotional pressure' of managing the COVID epidemic, an inquest was told. Vernon Hough, 61, ran Gwastad Hall Nursing Home in Wrexham, Wales, with his wife, Helen, caring for forty residents. He was found dead at a local police station car park on 21 May. His wife explained to the inquest how he had lost weight due to worrying about the pandemic, leading the coroner to conclude suicide was the cause of death.

Mrs Hough said running the care home meant that 'he was panicked … We would constantly talk about COVID-19 … he wasn't afraid of catching it, he was afraid of spreading it because we weren't being tested. That's what his fear was.' She described her husband as a 'worrier' who had lost 1.5 stone (9.5 kg) in weight 'due to the worry of Covid'.

Mr Hough had previously been prescribed anti-depressants by a GP, but it is clear to me that this tragic case exemplifies the continuing and enduring fiasco of the healthcare system failing to properly advise on and deal with, in the correct granular detail, these central issues of worry and panic. It is striking how often this poor man's wife mentioned the word 'worry' in her testimony to the inquest, yet how this core aspect of the case appeared to have been ignored by all those supposed to have been helping this man with his stress. He had clearly never been informed about the worry timetable technique nor the importance of 'clearing the attic', as discussed in the brain scanning study in our preface.

Experimental psychologists discovered a long time ago that it was not so much ordeals like electric shocks during torture which damaged us mentally, but rather the administering of unpredictable punishments. We can learn to cope with even the most difficult predicaments, as long as we know they are coming.

The stress-reducing effect of predictability hinges on recognising safe periods between traumas. In other words, once animals or humans appreciated when no harm would happen, they found it easier to cope with shocks. Unpredictability undermined this, and if adversity could occur anytime, then even the duration between disturbances had become unsafe. Most stress does not occur in actual emergencies, but during the periods *in-between* traumatic events.

Brosschot, Verkuil and Thayer[1] point out in their research paper that it is vital to recall that before the pandemic, stress was also unavoidable in life. Even those with superior coping skills have to confront the reality that there are always threats coming over the horizon. Disease and pain cannot be abolished, misfortune will keep threatening us incessantly. The vicious boss is unlikely to change, just as lions will always be present in the life of antelopes.

There is no vaccine for life.

To maintain good mental health, it is therefore vital to restrict our distress responses to when bad events are happening. The secret is to create as many safe periods as possible (without resorting to Class A drugs), even if this is something we need to do in our heads.

As an example, the authors cite the example of the antelope that never runs further away from the lion (the ever-present stressor) than necessary, allowing for adequate time to escape from the next attack: the safe zone.

Given the new central importance accorded to territoriality and the mental security implicit in 'safe places' by this new theory of stress, anxiety, worry, fear and panic, it is particularly intriguing that the very latest research finds anti-depressants transforming the feelings of wildlife about their turf.[16] A recent study involved injecting fluoxetine (Prozac is the brand, fluoxetine is the generic title for the same chemical) into sparrows, discovering that the birds became more chilled about defending their territory from other birds.[16] In other words, they seemed to feel safer within their terrain and had less need to be aggressive to neighbours. Another way of thinking about the essential effect of anti-depressants is that they make you feel you 'snug'. The identical outcome occurred after giving the same drug, Prozac, to coral reef fish. That study was entitled 'Fluoxetine treatment decreases territorial aggression in a coral reef fish'.[17]

If you could mentally feel more secure – whether that be a mental or physical space – maybe you wouldn't need anti-depressant drugs, as proved in these two recent studies injecting fluoxetine (Prozac) into sparrows and fish.

'What triggers anxiety?' is the wrong question.[18] The stress response, from an evolutionary perspective, is built into us to help us survive a precarious prairie. Instead, a better question is: 'What stops stress?' The answer is *safety*. Even if it is merely perceived shelter.

Animals don't worry, though they do get anxious; they handle their anxiety in a particular way, often better than us. We can learn from them to find secure territory too. But in order to do this, we may end up defining safety in a different way to our leaders. It could be that we decide that not visiting elderly relatives, not sending our children to school, or not opening the economy, is more dangerous than the official advice acknowledges.

However, we also know it cannot be the case that the world is perennially perilous, precisely because we're alive.

In fact, could you just check your pulse right now? Because, if you believed everything you are told about how dicey it is out there, if you can find a heartbeat, proving you are indeed still alive, it's a bit of a mystery how you survive the Russian roulette of every breath.

Always ask yourself, when facing the next crisis or emotional disturbance, what would an antelope do?

2

HOW TO PANIC PROPERLY
OVER THE PANDEMIC

How the wrong kind of panic can be as lethal as a virus, and what would Captain Sully do?

On 17 February 2003, a panic stampede at Chicago's E2 nightclub was triggered when security guards used pepper spray to break up a fight. Many patrons believed terrorists were attacking, so 1,500 simultaneously tried to escape. At the exit, people were knocked over and trampled by the ensuing crush. The pile of bodies reached six feet high. Twenty-one victims died from compressional asphyxiation.

Analysing examples such as these, Anthony Mawson,[1] Professor of Public Health at Jackson State University, USA, has written an analysis entitled 'Understanding Mass Panic and Other Collective Responses to Threat and Disaster', which argues that experts may have fundamentally misunderstood the panic reaction. Mawson's analysis predicts that behind the scenes, governments were terrified that mass hysteria and panic would become endemic following COVID-19.

The collective response to threatened disaster is usually predicted to be alarm, hysteria, and the breakdown of social order. This appears to be a natural reaction to physical danger and entrapment. But Mawson argues that instead of running away from danger because of panic, we tend to react to a threat by seeking to affiliate with others. We run toward the familiar because it appears safe. Yet many governmental anti-viral measures, from all over the world, produced social isolation, and a sense of entrapment, which is in fact more likely to be the source of anxiety, agitation and distress.

Mawson's analysis of research into the evacuation behaviour of occupants of the former World Trade Center following the explosion on 26 February 1993 is based on interviews with 350 participants. Those with the deepest social ties with others in the building were the slowest to begin evacuating.

Mawson cites further evidence that during the bombing raids on London in the Second World War, children displayed remarkably little distress, even if exposed to extremely violent scenes, if they were with a parent. It was only if children were separated from their families that serious psychological disturbances ensued. Disruption of the familial bond appeared more traumatic than air raids.

Officials experience great difficulty persuading people to evacuate before catastrophes; family ties often keep individuals in the danger zone until it's too late. Most residents remain in disaster areas, and those who escape early tend to be unattached to the locale. When residents are forced to evacuate, they tend to flee as a group.

A major panic gripping large numbers can also be ignited by a seemingly minor event – hundreds and even thousands of troops can turn and run in panic from the front line of battle after witnessing just one soldier running away. Perhaps this is explained as the initial bolting being experienced by the observer as a threat to social ties, and as signalling abandonment and separation. The subsequent action of the observer is not an attempt to escape danger but an effort to maintain proximity with those who started escaping.

Panic is an affiliative response.

In certain situations, such as fires in buildings, the tendency to seek the familiar in the face of imminent physical danger can have disastrous consequences. Ironically, because tendencies toward hysteria and mass panic on the part of the public are widely assumed, Mawson argues that officials are often reluctant to issue warnings, or delay doing so, for fear of igniting a stampede. Yet delays in providing correct sufficient information can result in entrapment and death due to inactivity. The problem during disasters is not that people tend to get scared and act impulsively in response to danger, but that they delay, failing to take evasive action when it is urgently needed.

Despite all the behavioural expertise supposedly available to governments, the population experienced unprecedented panic during the pandemic.

These are the suggestive results of new research using internet searches as a clue to the mental state of citizens. An academic study[2] just published in the *Journal of the American Medical Association – Internal Medicine* analysed a precipitous rise in internet searches using terms like 'panic attack' and 'anxiety attack' in the early days of the pandemic's arrival in the USA. The investigation found that on one day, 28 March 2020, shortly after social distancing was first introduced, internet searches for such terms spiked, reaching 52 per cent more queries than would be expected during an equivalent 'normal' period. The team of researchers monitored the daily fraction of all internet searches that included the terms 'anxiety' or 'panic' in combination with 'attack' (including 'panic attack', 'signs of anxiety attack', 'anxiety attack symptoms') originating from the USA between 1 January 2004 and 4 May 2020.

The study found all acute anxiety queries were 11 per cent higher than expected for the fifty-eight-day period that started when President Trump first declared a national emergency (13 March 2020) and ended with the last available date of data (9 May 2020). This spike was an all-time high for acute anxiety searches, translating to approximately 375,000 more searches than expected.

Moreover, most excess queries occurred between 16 March and 14 April, when queries were cumulatively 17 per cent higher than expected. During this time, national social distancing guidelines were first imposed (16 March 2020) and extended (29 March 2020), the USA passed China with the most reported cases (26 March 2020), the Centres for Disease Control and Prevention recommended using facemasks (3 April 2020), and the USA passed Italy for most deaths (11 April 2020).

Although this study cannot confirm that any search was linked to a specific acute anxiety event or panic attack, the authors argue that it provides evidence for psychological effects arising from COVID-19 because our internet searches do reveal something about our mental state.

Mawson argues that under a variety of stressful conditions, individuals approach familiar persons and places and are calmed by their presence. There is an increase in 'we-feeling', solidarity and morale, but also a parallel increased sensitivity to perceived deviance and a tendency toward social exclusion, scapegoating, and hate crime.

Officialdom has failed to understand the essential nature of panic, a fiercely strong emotion which is not about running *away* from something, which is maybe what they wanted us to do from COVID-19. Instead, acute anxiety involves running *toward* the familiar and protection, with an urge for group solidarity.

Imposing social isolation after terrifying the population may have been particularly damaging for mental health, and for the effectiveness of quarantining, because officials failed to grasp the ultimate true purpose of panic. The public were scared to death, and then on top of that were told to keep away from each other. The 'screws', to use prison parlance for those in charge, as a result, screwed everyone up.

On 18 August, *The Daily Telegraph* reported[3] that UK Government figures show people who live alone are twice as likely to test positive for coronavirus, with 'experts', the newspaper reported, claiming it is 'more difficult' for them to remain isolated.

As those in charge don't understand how people react to panic, their directives result in people ending up in precisely the opposite place to where they should be, such as at the top of a burning tower block, rather than the bottom (see the next chapter on the Grenfell Tower disaster). Or, in a lockdown, they end up being much more sociable than it is safe to be.

This fundamental failure of our government to grasp how the public really feel and then how they act was indeed similar to the essential error wartime authorities made in trying to get Londoners to take refuge from the Luftwaffe bombing campaign in air-raid shelters and underground stations. Wartime authorities believed the public would naturally take refuge in the official shelters as advised. But they got this badly wrong. Some bomb shelters were even eventually closed because of low occupancy.

A study entitled 'The psychology of protecting the UK public against external threat: COVID-19 and the Blitz compared'[4] contends that in November 1940 of the 3.2 million people living in inner London only 4 per cent took shelter in underground railway stations. That old black-and-white wartime footage of hundreds cowering on tube platforms in an apparent act of solidarity gives a completely false impression of what really happened. Some 5 per cent occupied street shelters, while 27 per cent slept in garden air-raid structures. Most people (64 per cent) remained home during the aerial bombardment. They preferred the feeling of safety derived from loved ones in a familiar environment. Rationally, that was probably more dangerous than retreating to the underground.

People have this stubborn tendency to surprise their leaders and the experts advising them, which also explains why modelling, which depends on predicting human behaviour, has so often landed wide of the mark. Governments have a long and undistinguished history of being completely off beam in their analysis of how people process threat.

Another, better, way of thinking about the nature of panic in any predicament is always to ask yourself, when not sure what to do – for example, whether to panic or not – what would Captain Sully do?

Captain Chesley (Sully) Sullenberger was piloting US Airways Flight 1549 in January 2009 when he was forced to ditch in the Hudson River. The 'Miracle on the Hudson' is the focus of the 2016 blockbuster Tom Hanks movie *Sully*. Sully's plane collided with birds almost immediately after take-off, producing dramatic engine power loss.

Leon Assael, Dean of the School of Dentistry, University of Minnesota, USA, writing in an academic journal for surgeons and attempting to glean lessons for doctors who must demonstrate similar unflappability in emergencies, comments: 'The flight recording of the final 2.5 minutes of Flight 1549 are extraordinary in the coolness and business-like words of Sully, ending with "Teterboro no good ... We'll be in the Hudson."'

In his study he asks whether, given 'Sully' Sullenberger achieved what no pilot had ever done before – crashing a commercial jet on water without the loss of life – are there lessons for all of us struggling to be similarly heroic within our own personal crises?

> Sully calmly spent what was likely the last 2.5 minutes of his life working with his co-pilot going through the engine restart checklist, assessing his navigation to optimise the best place to ditch, communicating with the Westbury control tower, managing his crew and passengers, lifting the nose, barely clearing the mid-span of the George Washington Bridge, missing the boats in the harbour, dropping his tail to impact the water first, hydroplaning to a stop, safely evacuating all passengers and crew, assessing that his plane was empty of all souls, and then leading his crew in the water rescue of every single passenger.[5]

What the Hollywood depiction of heroism misses, however, is that Sully and the flight crew all suffered from trauma symptoms for many months afterwards. Dr Marjorie Podraza Stiegler[6] from the Anesthesiology Department, University of North Carolina at Chapel Hill, USA, in a study entitled 'What I Learned About Adverse Events From Captain Sully – It's Not What You Think', asks why,

... if Captain Sully's years of experience had all been a cumulative preparation for this most unlikely event, and if he did just about everything right (and quickly), could he not sleep or concentrate for three months? Why did he need medications to control his racing heart and high blood pressure? Why could he not return to the skies for nearly half a year? First Officer Jeff Skiles experienced similar aftermath, according to Sully ... even the air traffic controller Patrick Harten had to be removed immediately from duty and was unable to return to work for about a month and reported only beginning to feel good about that event a full year later. Mr Harten says, 'It may sound strange, but for me the hardest part of the event was when it was over. During the event I was hyper-focused ... but when it was over, it hit me hard.' Captain Sully shared this sentiment, telling me that he felt in control during the event, and in shock immediately afterwards, and the total impact took some time to process. The flight crew also took time away, and one flight crew member with 38 years of experience never returned. I was surprised to know that after a hugely successful demonstration of teamwork and skill, and a landmark safety save, all of the parties involved were so adversely affected.

Leon Assae points out:

When asked during an interview if he panicked or prayed during those final moments, Sully seemed surprised by the question. 'Why no,' he replied. 'There were plenty of people in the back of the plane doing that for me... But afterwards, I really let go.'

Perhaps one answer to the conundrum of how to confront anxiety and terror is that during an emergency, heroes focus on what needs to be done to survive, or save lives.[7] This means they are able to shove panic to one side, preventing interference with survival. But when the immediate crisis is over, maybe it is the lack of an immediately pressing goal which releases the underlying emotional turmoil. Once the urgency is over, there is no remaining imperative to suppress feelings.[8]

Maybe the process isn't helped by all those well-meaning friends, relatives and even counsellors constantly inquiring, 'How are you feeling?' After all, no one in Sully's cockpit checked whether anyone 'wanted to share' in the seconds before diving into the Hudson.

In surviving acute adversity, emotions take the back seat while the brain takes command of the careening vehicle that is your life.

This suggests that in order to overcome anxiety and fear you need a pressing resolve or reason which will help you suppress emotion, not ventilate it. Most anxious and fearful people are encouraged to share their feelings, and are waiting to become less tense before pursuing goals.[9] It could be that precisely the opposite strategy is what is required; hunt for objectives, and then you will feel better. Pursue goals despite the fact your emotions are not set up for them. The pilot crash-landing the plane in which you're travelling doesn't get on the intercom to explain that they'll address the emergency once their emotions have returned to equilibrium.

There is a sense in which the everyday bravery of ordinary folk is vastly underrated, because Hollywood has convinced us heroism means skimming a jet over water. Yet millions crawl out of bed, and not to a Hollywood star's luxurious life; instead, every day, they suppress horrendous, unpleasant emotions, just to turn up to some mind-numbing job that feels like crawling through barbed wire.

The pandemic, through lockdowns, suddenly deprived us of the everyday goals (like getting to work) that routinely levered us out of bed in the morning, helping us shove negative emotions to one side. When those reasons evaporate, we have to discover our own daily purpose. If we don't, then negative emotions will invade, occupying swathes of territory in our mental landscape, strangling our ability to govern ourselves.

Maybe one lesson from the story of Sully is that courage is more ordinary than extraordinary. Perhaps we are all more capable of heroism than the Hollywood depiction of the 'heroic' allows?

The goal that gets you out of bed in the morning doesn't have to be grand or impressive, like saving lives on a crashing aeroplane; it could be simply to go for a run, which is better for you than staying in bed all day. To do this is, in a sense, a form of heroism.

In the chapter entitled 'Resilience' in the *Encyclopedia of Mental Health* is the following:[10] 'The regularity with which humans overcome life obstacles has been referred to as "ordinary magic" ... a notion that contradicts much popular press coverage of "overcoming the odds".'

Leon Assael references Ralph Waldo Emerson, who declared: 'A hero is no braver than an ordinary man, but he is braver five minutes longer.'

3

LIVING WITH LOSS DURING LOCKDOWN

Does the Grenfell Tower tragedy reveal how to live with loss during lockdown?

On 14 June 2017, a conflagration ravaged the twenty-four-storey Grenfell Tower block of flats in North Kensington, West London. The resulting seventy-two deaths ensured this became the deadliest fire within a structure in the United Kingdom since the 1988 Piper Alpha disaster, and the most devastating UK residential fire since the Second World War. One of the enduring controversies is exactly why most of those killed were said to have been between the eleventh and twenty-third floors.[1]

One theory is that some from lower floors may have moved *up* the building, and there were rumours that a large number of victims ended up in one room, where they met what must be one of the most horrifying ends it is possible to imagine. Firefighters described finding finding eight people from various flats who had congregated in one apartment on the fourteenth floor. Emergency workers at the inquiry appeared surprised that so many should have come together from different flats to this one, and there was also confusion over how to get such a large number down. The final moments of some of the residents in that particular apartment were recalled by firefighter Christopher Batchelor, speaking at the inquiry.[1] It was a horrifying description.

A better understanding of the panic response in emergency scenarios from which large numbers need to escape could help prevent these kinds of tragedies happening in the future.

There is a very strong tendency for people to move towards each other for safety, as opposed to fleeing from each other to the outside. Yet this new understanding has not featured in the subsequent inquiries, nor in any psychological analysis to understand human behaviour during this most panicky of tragedies.

Nor has it informed current lockdown restrictions.

Another heart-rending aspect of the West London tower block fire was the plight of relatives and friends, beside themselves with anxiety and worry over the fate of the missing in the hours and days immediately following the cataclysm. Is trying to cope with uncertainty about the fate of a missing person the very worst kind of grief? This particularly dreadful predicament is referred to by experts as 'ambiguous loss' because it remains unclear what has definitively happened to the missing person; the psychology of hope is naturally activated.

The workings of ambiguous loss are particularly pertinent to surviving the pandemic; many of the deprivations are indeed uncertain. You are not sure if you are going to see elderly relatives ever again, nor whether your industry is going to recover and see you get your job back.

Hope becomes a double-edged sword, inspiring at times, engendering a desire to keep fighting on – but if or when hope is dashed, perhaps even deeper despair follows. It is this turmoil of contrasting emotions, endlessly oscillating between hope and despair, which renders coping particularly stressful, and may prevent the achivement of 'closure' or mental peace. In ambiguous loss, it is the hope that ends up destroying you. Which is worse: to know definitively that a loved one has been killed, or not to know what happened save that someone has gone missing?

A study[2] recently investigated this precise question. The research compared the impact on two groups of women living in Bosnia and Herzegovina: those whose husbands were confirmed as having been killed during the 1992–95 war, and those whose husbands were still listed as missing as a result of the conflict.

The researchers found the group with unconfirmed losses had higher levels of traumatic grief as well as severe depression. The authors concluded that this group's particularly high levels of severe depression, including suicidal thinking, were especially worrying.

Another recent study entitled 'When hope and grief intersect: Rates and risks of prolonged grief disorder among bereaved individuals and relatives of disappeared persons in Colombia'[3] compared those who lost a significant other simply by their 'disappearance' against the straightforwardly bereaved. It found the extent of hope in those dealing with a disappearance predicted 'Prolonged Grief Disorder'.

Prolonged Grief Disorder is referred to by the authors of this study[3] as a grief reaction following loss, characterised by intense longing and yearning for the lost person, combined with feelings of hopelessness and emptiness over a period of at least six months. The study found the more strongly people hope that their loved one is still alive, the greater the severity of Prolonged Grief Disorder symptoms.

For various reasons it is likely that COVID-19 will be a major cause of Prolonged Grief Disorder.

Psychologists have attempted to study how to best counsel those suffering in this predicament and some have argued against delivering 'false hope'. Yet some would-be rescuers did just that in the acutely stressful environment at Grenfell Tower; and perhaps in those particular circumstances such a course of action was not unreasonable. It may be that there is a balance to be struck between trying to counsel against unrealistic or unjustifiable levels of hopefulness and simply crushing all hope.

While it may seem blindingly obvious what people are hoping for – the person being alive and well – this faith may nevertheless evolve over time, for example, into praying that the missing person did not suffer. The problem is that while the hope persists, it leads to incessant dwelling upon the missing person, interfering with daily life, leading to collapse in the long run.

We have become used to images of missing people posted on street corners as signifying the hope of those searching for any news, and this phenomenon seems to have first been studied as a coping mechanism following the 9/11 tragedy in New York. It may be that this is the kind of heartbreak where, uniquely, hope makes you worse.

How does psychiatric practice help us with our tragic but ultimately unavoidable losses? Many psychologists contend that 'ambiguous loss' is a lot more common than realised. For example, when a loved one develops severe dementia, they remain physically present, but have in a sense also 'gone missing', in terms of the person you once knew.

Viktor Frankl, a famous psychiatrist who survived the Holocaust, argued there can be no meaning to our lives without hope, and no hope without meaning. Viktor Frankl lived and worked among those for whom there could surely be no hope, as they had lost everything, and knew they were going to be killed. Yet he contended it was possible to find meaning in our lives even in the face of the most brutal and inhuman catastrophe, as he himself had directly experienced at the hands of the Nazis.

The art of survival would appear to hinge on how to find new meaning and hope in life, according to Frankl, and this might mean having to say goodbye even when you remain uncertain over the fate of your loved one. This sometimes feels like a betrayal.

With any ambiguous loss, you are the one who has to make the choice to finally say goodbye; whereas in every other kind of bereavement, that decision is forced upon you. But the fact that the victim of ambiguous loss must have experienced love and attachment – for grief is the heavy price we pay for love – is also maybe something on which we can base our hope for the future, because that love made life worthwhile.

The very reason for the despair is the foundation of our hopes for the future.

Coping with such severe losses or traumas will never be easy. However, to simplify how it can be achieved, psychiatrists divide this coping into four main tasks of grieving, or successful bereavement.

The 'Four Task' model of coping with loss is an extremely powerful tool, yet little discussed properly in the world of mental health. Instead, most counsellors seem to favour a much better known yet much less helpful model, which refers to phases of grief during a loss. This is an inferior approach because it emphasises passivity on the part of anyone grieving. The 'Four Task' model in contrast is much more active and insists that you have to go and do something – in fact a series of things, hence the four tasks – in order to recover successfully from loss.

Given the pandemic involves multiple losses for many people, the 'Four Task' model is right at the centre of coping with COVID-19. These losses include possibly a cessation of income or unemployment, relationship breakdown, or even just missing a normal social life.

That ambiguous loss may be particularly difficult is exemplified by the story of Sir Patrick Stewart, one of the most distinguished actors of his generation, most well known for playing Captain Jean-luc Picard in the Star Trek film franchise.[4] The eminent Shakespearian actor confided in *The Daily Telegraph* in aid of Refuge, the domestic abuse charity, that he had been in therapy for two decades. This seemed a bit of a surprise given how much confidence must be involved in live theatre performance, as well as having all those cameras trained on you.

But during a West Yorkshire childhood of grinding poverty in the 1940s and 1950s, he regularly directly witnessed extreme violence meted out by his father on his defenceless mother.

This so traumatised him that Sir Patrick Stewart, at the age of eighty, was still in weekly psychotherapy and had been for the previous twenty years.

But perhaps the key trauma was not knowing on any one particular evening if his father was going to turn violent, and so the ordeal was deeply unpredictable. Given his mother also always refused to leave her abusive husband despite the entreaties of her children, including young Patrick, the trauma perhaps remained in some sense ambiguous.

Given his neighbour heard the violence but did nothing, perhaps another ambiguity was, given their silence, whether anything truly terrible was really happening. It must have been very confusing for a child and all the more harrowing. He confided to Guy Kelly of *The Daily Telegraph*:

> We became experts at knowing when the moment had arrived in the shouting when we had to physically put our bodies between our mother and our father. Children should not [have to] become experts at this kind of thing, but we knew when violence was about to happen because we'd seen it so many times ... I knew that all of our neighbours knew what happened in our house, and it humiliated me, shamed me. My brother and I felt ourselves responsible for what happened, but of course we were not. To know that you were surrounded by people who were aware of the horror stayed with me, and that's why I never talked about it.

Whenever anyone appears 'stuck' in therapy it might be that they are wrestling with some aspect of ambiguous loss, so that instead of endless therapeutic 'sharing', they need another survival strategy. Perhaps Sir Patrick, and many others, could have avoided twenty years of weekly therapy if he had been aware of the 'Four Task' model of coping with loss.

The model includes both the idea of the work a person must do in order to cope with their loss, as well as the sequence in which the activities should be carried out – the first task being completed before moving on to the second, and so on.

The model also helps to pinpoint the stage where someone may have become stuck, which explains why they continue to suffer excessively, despite appearing to have been appropriately dealing with it.

This notion that the tasks have to be done in particular order is an extremely powerful aspect of this model because it provides a direct guide as to what to do and when while recovering from loss. You can also backtrack to discover which task may not have been accomplished correctly to ascertain where a misstep could have been made if you are stuck at any one point.

The Four Tasks are:

(1) Accept the Reality of the Loss
(2) Ventilate the Emotions
(3) Learn New Skills
(4) Re-invest the Emotions.

Note the very precise terminology, and this is also an extremely important aspect of the Four Task model. We don't say just 'accept the loss', instead we insist on 'accept the REALITY of the loss'.

What do these terms mean and how are we to implement them?

The first task of grieving is to accept the reality of the loss. Many of the recently bereaved behave as if their loved one is still alive. They may lay a place at the table for them, or even hallucinate that they are around. Or, like Dickens's Miss Havisham, they keep their rotting wedding dress on show. In the early stages of a loss, this behaviour is so common as to be considered almost a normal part of grieving. But if it is still going on many months after the death, it shows that the loss has not been fully accepted.

The term 'reality of the loss' applies to many situations other than just the loss of a person. It applies, for example, to the pushy parents whose child fails at exams, and who need to accept the loss of their ambitions for their child to excel at school. If Victor Meldrew ever started to say, 'I do believe it,' it would show that he had begun to accept the deprivation.

After accepting, intellectually, the reality of the loss, the second task of grieving is to release and deal with the emotions that follow from this acceptance. These may range from anger to frustration or despair. Whatever they are, acknowledging and expressing them is extremely important.

In my experience those who make a poor recovery from deep loss often appear on the outside to have coped magnificently, organising the funeral or busying themselves with a hobby. Yet, because they have never articulated their hurt, be it as despair, anger or even relief, these moods will never have been dealt with. They will therefore contribute to longer-lasting problems which may not emerge until years later. If we do not express how we feel, particularly with disturbing emotions, an important part of us is unacknowledged. This disregard contributes to a growing feeling of alienation between us and others or even between us and our true selves.

Once this second task has been completed, the third task can be attempted, that of learning new skills.

Whenever we suffer a fundamental loss, it usually means we will have to adapt to it and this may require additional competencies. Those who have lost a partner who was good at filling out forms and following recipes may have to learn how to manage the finances or how to cook. The parents of our unacademic child may have to learn how to play with their offspring rather than constantly push them academically, and so on. If you have become unemployed, coping with the loss of a job may mean learning the new skills of occupying yourself during the day, budgeting and facing up to the loss of status when socialising.

Those who have not accepted the reality of the loss – task number one – may have particular difficulty seeing the need for new skills as they feel the latest situation is more temporary than it really is. It is difficult to start the onerous task of learning new skills if you are still bogged down with the need to articulate emotions produced by the loss, or are struggling to accept the reality of the loss. But once tasks one and two are completed, new skills need to be acquired; otherwise coping will be stuck here.

Once the third task has been completed, the fourth and final task beckons. This is to reinvest into some new project the emotional energy that was allotted to the person or thing that has been lost. Those who have lost a partner may have to reinvest their feelings into someone else – another partner, friend or relative – or perhaps become engaged in charity work.

You may recall from the introduction how the family of Lorna Breen, that eminent head of the hospital emergency department, had started a charity devoted to the mental health of clinicians. This is a more central part of the better way of coping with grief and loss than might be realised. This is Task Four in action. The way the press reported the story it looked like it was just an incidental occurrence following the death of the doctor.

It is also notable that, as suggested by the Four Task model, the other three tasks had to be accomplished first before number four could be finally implemented successfully, and this may explain why this fourth task was being initiated a few months following the funeral.

Of course, if a loss is fundamental enough, there may be no way you can replace it; but there has to be some attempt to fill the emotional hole left. When one of Freud's children split up with a suitor whom she had hoped to marry, the astute psychiatrist, aware of the need to complete task four to recover from a loss, bought his 'mourning' daughter a pet dog. Having someone to look after and dote on, and which in turn reciprocated her feelings of affection, cured the forlorn child of lovesickness. Nowadays, pets are even formally recommended as part of the treatment for grief.

One very interesting implication of the Four Task model of coping with loss is that at no point does it mention counselling or therapy. What it is proposing is that it is entirely possible to cope successfully with loss whether you do the tasks inside therapy or outside it.

This is an essential point, as it means that coping with COVID-19 doesn't mean you need to go and see a therapist.

Was a version of the fourth task, of 're-investing the emotions', being accomplished by Sir Patrick Stewart in supporting the domestic abuse charity Refuge as a way of making peace with his feeling that he hadn't done enough to protect his mother from his father? Might that be a better way of processing the loss of his mother than therapy?

In fact, bereavement counselling – long considered by psychologists to be vital in recovering from the death of a loved one – may be more of a waste of time than is commonly realised. There have been challenges to the belief in its efficacy, which has been firmly held by psychoanalysts since Sigmund Freud proposed in 1917 that confronting feelings is the healthiest way to cope with bereavement. Many psychoanalysts have even argued that failure to express grief indicates – or may lead to – deep psychological problems. Bereavement counsellors often urge people to express their sadness in order to release 'suppressed emotions'. However, a group of psychologists from Utrecht University in the Netherlands who carried out their own research and reviewed that of others has found no link between emotional expression of grief and a diminution of subsequent distress.[5] They assessed 128 recently bereaved people four times over two years and found no significant statistical difference between the continued distress in those who shared their emotions and those who did not.

The authors also challenged the view that it is beneficial for those who have suffered loss to 'write about their very deepest thoughts and feelings'. They reviewed previous trials in which bereaved people had been asked to write for fifteen to thirty minutes either about a recent traumatic loss or a trivial topic, and found little evidence that writing about emotions was beneficial.

Do you recall the advice from the Introduction of that BBC doctor about making a list? The authors of this investigation commented: 'The findings challenge beliefs about grief work, emotional disclosure and beneficial interventions that were considered as self-evident by bereavement researchers only a decade ago.'

They concluded that the most common difficulty suffered by bereaved people is emotional loneliness: the feeling of being utterly alone, even when in the company of friends and family. This type of loneliness, they say, only abates with time and nothing can be done to aid recovery.

The findings are supported by Dr Colin Murray Parkes,[5] a consultant psychiatrist and the president of the charity Cruse Bereavement Care:

> There is no evidence that all bereaved people will benefit from counselling, and research has shown no benefit to arise from the routine referral of people to counselling for no other reason than that they have suffered bereavement.

Yet Prince Harry has recently revealed that he had been in therapy for seven years to cope with the death of his mother. In February 2020 Prince Harry[6] spoke openly and movingly about how he coped with the death of his mother, Princess Diana. Childhood parental death is regarded by psychologists as one of the most severely stressful life events that a child can experience. Did what Harry said reveal an indispensable secret which might help others deal with the multiplicity of losses inflicted by the pandemic? Losing a parent during childhood is such a major event: surely if there are coping strategies that assist with overcoming this trauma, they might help the rest of us survive the losses wreaked by COVID-19?

In the United States, at any given time, 3.5 per cent of the population, or roughly 2.2 million people, have endured the death of one or both of their parents prior to reaching the age of eighteen; in the UK it is 4 to 5 per cent.[7]

The coping mechanism which has been found to be one of the most powerful in promoting resilience in childhood survivors of parental death was also recently uncovered in survivors of the 9/11 attacks in the USA.

Nathan Greene and Katie McGovern have published a study of 350 adults who experienced early parental death in order to investigate which coping skills best assist psychological survival. This study, entitled 'Gratitude, psychological well-being, and perceptions of post-traumatic growth in adults who lost a parent in childhood',[8] points out that following the 9/11 attacks psychological research into those who appeared more psychologically resilient suggested they might have been deploying the coping skill of gratitude.

The pivotal factor referred to as 'dispositional gratitude' is strongly associated with psychological well-being and post-traumatic growth, even if you lost a parent during childhood. This tendency to feel grateful for what life has to offer, despite the bad hand of cards you seem to have been dealt, also protected against developing depression.

Psychologists had already found from their surveys that grateful people tend to be happier, but is this an attitude to life that can be learned, practised and cultivated?[9] Or are you just born that way? Well, it has been found that gratitude and well-being *do* increase when following techniques such as maintaining a gratitude journal or actively counting one's blessings.[10]

Gratitude was one of the three most reported positive emotions from those traumatised by the attacks, and these people may have felt grateful to be alive or to know that their loved ones were safe.

The most common reason given in Greene and McGovern's study for experiencing no change or a decrease in gratitude was that the emotional pain related to the loss was too great to allow for thankfulness. Many reported that difficulty trusting others, resentment and family conflict inhibited what they called gratitude formation.

In their study, however, the counter-intuitive finding is that such a profoundly negative experience as losing a parent during childhood can lead you to feel more gratitude or appreciation for life because of a newfound belief that life is precious, with greater appreciation for loved ones. Witnessing first-hand the death of a parent at a young age could lead one to view life as a finite commodity, and in turn to value one's own life more as well as the lives of others. As one participant in this research reported:

I know and understand very much how short life can be and how the important people in our lives might only be here for a short amount of time. I take each day as an opportunity to do things that are meaningful to me and try to find ways to connect with the people I care about.

4

COULD THE PANDEMIC RESULT IN 50,000 SUICIDES WORLDWIDE? HOW NOT TO BECOME JUST ANOTHER STATISTIC

Latest research finds some suicidal people may try to catch COVID-19 on purpose

The Golden Gate Bridge in San Francisco is regarded as one of the most beautiful structures in the world, and is perhaps one of the most photographed. In 1937, just three months after the popular tourist destination first opened, it began its journey to becoming famous for an altogether much more sinister reason.

H. B. Wobber, a forty-nine-year-old bargeman, looking like any other tourist in August, took a coach to the popular sightseeing destination, and began strolling across the mile-long span. Appearing to be enjoying the view, he chatted to a Professor Louis Nailer of Trinity College in Connecticut, a fellow tourist he'd just met on the bus. They'd ambled across the full span, which reaches in a single sweeping arch from San Francisco to the hills of Marin County, and were returning to the pedestrian turnstile from which they had first entered, when Wobber unexpectedly tossed his coat and outer vest to the professor.

'This is where I get off,' he said softly. 'I'm going to jump.' As Wobber clambered over the 4-foot barrier, the professor managed to grasp his belt, but Wobber struggled free and vaulted to his death. Since then, it is thought that more than 2,000 others have jumped, making it the world's number one location for suicide.

One theory as to why the bridge is such a popular destination for the hopeless and despairing is the widely held, yet mistaken, belief that a dive from the beautifully serene bridge is calm, rapid and fatal. It is calculated that if you do jump you hit the water at 75 miles an hour, with the 200-foot fall lasting 4 seconds. Jumpers therefore die from massive cardiothoracic and brain injuries.[1] Even if the impact doesn't kill the victim, the fierce current will sweep the dazed or stunned victim out to sea to drown, or to be devoured by sharks.

Doctors Mel Blaustein and Anne Fleming[1] published a study of suicides from this bridge, ascertaining that thirty people have survived the jump. They report of one survivor:

> Intent on suicide, he tearfully bypassed the phones [suicide prevention phones offering counselling that have been placed on the bridge given the high suicide rate] but told himself that if one person showed concern he would not jump. When a German tourist approached him but requested only that he take her picture, he complied, muttered under his breath, walked away, then threw himself over the railing. He later reported how thankful he was to be alive, confirming that many suicides are impulsive and preventable.

Dr John Jacobs read their article and sent this letter[2] in response to the *American Journal of Psychiatry*:

> A few years ago, I visited the Golden Gate Bridge and took a picture (Figure 1). The sign at the edge of the bridge read as follows: 'Emergency Phone and Crisis Counselling.' Under the sign was a telephone wrapped in yellow CAUTION tape with the words 'Out of Order'.

Death by suicide is estimated to occur every eleven minutes in the US, and a new form of self-harm might be emerging: seeking to catch COVID-19 *on purpose*.

This is the startling conclusion of a study entitled 'Preliminary Investigation of the Association Between COVID-19 and Suicidal Thoughts and Behaviors in the US'.[3] This survey found that some individuals in the USA may be intentionally exposing themselves to the virus, with the intention of killing themselves. The authors of the study point out in their paper that before the COVID-19 pandemic, it was recognised that suicidal people may attempt to contract diseases, for example HIV, as a method of dying.

This is the first study to examine the link between COVID-19 and suicidal thoughts and behaviours, as well as to explore intentional COVID-19 exposure. The research found that eighty-three US adults (9.2 per cent of their sample) reported intentionally exposing themselves to COVID-19. Given how contagious the virus is, the authors contend this has enormous public health implications.

The reasons these people gave for seeking to intentionally expose themselves to the virus included 'Wanted a break from life', 'Wanted to punish self', 'Wanted to hurt self (without wanting to die)', 'Didn't want to be alive anymore' and 'Wanted to kill self'. Of note, approximately 50 per cent who intentionally exposed themselves indicated their reason for doing so was 'strongly-to-extremely' due to wanting to kill themselves.

As the epidemic continues to spread, those suffering severe psychological distress will gain increased access to a potentially lethal means of suicide. The authors of this study conclude there is an urgent need to investigate to what extent intentional self-exposure to COVID-19, possibly borne of suicidal intent, might be spreading across the USA.

This study found that upwards of 45 per cent of individuals admitting to suicidal thinking in the previous month reported that their thoughts were explicitly linked to COVID-19 at least half of the time; indeed, approximately 65 per cent reported this to be the case at least some of the time.

The results suggest that the virus is having a direct negative effect on the mental health of the population and may be directly contributing to suicidal thinking.

But could the cure, in the form of 'lockdown' and all its restrictions, still be worse than the disease? Separate to the direct effect of the infection, what about the repercussions of the pandemic in terms of the economic and social consequences? Could the lockdown be making people suicidal more than the virus itself?

Following the last great recession of 2008 there was a dramatic increase in suicides in North America and Europe: an extra 10,000 people in those regions killed themselves between 2008 and 2010.

These shocking results came from a study[4] published in the *British Journal of Psychiatry* which demonstrated that, using statistical and comparison techniques, it was possible to confirm that the economic downturn had contributed to a raised suicide rate. The study also figured out what number of the additional suicides were linked to the recession. But whether the current pandemic is predicted to produce an economic meltdown of much greater breadth and depth than the recession of 2008, in at least some parts of the world, continues to hinge precariously on the fluctuating progress over vaccine roll-outs, competing with rises in virus variant numbers. How many more people might kill themselves as a direct result?

Authors from Iowa State University and Stanford University have conducted a study[5] which suggests that 50,000 extra suicides worldwide is currently the best estimate of the result of the current pandemic.

They point out that the forecast could be much higher depending upon the level of unemployment and its duration and the concomitant length of isolation, even potentially contributing to 100,000 extra suicides worldwide. The authors are keen to emphasise that their numbers are just a forecast; however, they urge that they be acted upon now with a view to vigorous prevention of such an outcome.

Their current forecast is for the raised suicide rate to endure for up to two years from now.

The authors[5] developed a statistical forecast using previous estimates of the impact of unemployment and social isolation on suicide rates from past published research. They then factored into their model the current predicted unemployment and social isolation data for the present pandemic.

The researchers included in their modelling the known stressful impacts of quarantine conditions, including post-traumatic stress symptoms, confusion, anger, infection fears, frustration, boredom, inadequate supplies and information, financial loss, and stigma contributing to psychological stress. Feelings of guilt may be also be common, associated with not performing normal work or parenting duties.

Previous research has established that loneliness was reported in 38.5 per cent and social isolation in 60.6 per cent of those quarantined during the 2003 severe acute respiratory syndrome (SARS) outbreak in Canada.

This new article cites other studies that find that those who have felt very lonely and isolated from other people in just the previous two weeks were subsequently three times more likely to feel highly suicidal. Other research has found that merely living alone doubles the risk of suicide for women; it also raises it in men, but not to the same extent.

This unprecedented lockdown has also removed, in a much more profound manner than any previous epidemic, possible compensatory supporting relationships from friends, family, neighbourhood, church, school and work. As a result, the researchers predict more than 35,000 additional suicides worldwide, solely owing to loneliness and isolation produced by the pandemic.

On top of these difficulties is layered the strain of unemployment. According to International Labour Organisation estimates, the pandemic could result in upwards of 24.7 million jobs being lost worldwide. According to the US National Longitudinal Mortality Study, unemployed men are twice as likely to commit suicide as those who are employed, with unemployed women 3.8 times more likely to kill themselves than their employed counterparts.

The researchers[5] just focused on social isolation, deleterious mental health consequences and unemployment, as these are well known to be major predictors for suicide. But given that there are also other implicated factors which they did not include, their estimates err on the conservative side.

Their conclusion is that, purely as a result of increased unemployment, the USA may experience over 3,800 additional suicides, and the world more than 5,100. Similarly, isolation and loneliness, they expect, will contribute over 5,600 additional suicides in the USA and more than 35,000 across the rest of the world. In total, this research predicts a very rough estimate of 50,000 extra suicides worldwide as a direct result of the current pandemic.

As these parameters change – say the unemployment rates turn out to be higher, or lockdown goes on for longer than anticipated – they point out that the eventual numbers could be much worse.

For example, a variable which may not have been fully accounted for in the latest modelling, because of its unprecedented nature, is that the sales of firearms (one of the most common and also most deadly of suicide methods) have been reaching record levels in the USA since the pandemic started. The authors[3] argue that it is therefore urgent for public mental health campaigns to reflect the increased suicide risk, now that the community has more access to guns.

All deaths have a devastating impact, of course, but it could be argued that suicide proves especially costly in human terms: it is so often those who are otherwise physically healthy, with many more years of active life ahead of them, who kill themselves. Dying through a mere mental impulse, when no physical disorder would have taken you instead, could be construed as being a much more 'unnecessary' death.

In contrast, it could be argued that people who die from causes like a viral illness which preferentially strikes the elderly or those with prior conditions are those who generally would have had fewer quality years left.

This may seem like a somewhat cold-blooded calculation. Yet it is, in a sense, the kind of balancing act our leaders – and we as a society – are making right now. The suicidal, given the stigma surrounding mental illness and suicidality, tend not to stand up for themselves and fight their corner as robustly as others affected by new governmental restrictions. They tend not to be on the streets demonstrating for the need to end the lockdown. Instead, suicidal depression leads to retreat, avoidance and inhibition.

In which case, publicising ominous research results like these becomes one way to help fight their corner for them.

Mark D. Griffiths, a psychologist at Nottingham Trent University, and Mohammed Mamun from the Department of Public Health & Informatics at Jahangirnagar University in Bangladesh have recently published an investigation with the disturbing finding[6] that it is possible the pandemic may be responsible for a rise in couples committing suicide and suicide pacts. Their reported case studies include:

An American couple from Lockport, Illinois – Patrick Jesernik (aged 54 years) and partner Cheryl Schriefer (aged 59) – were involved in a COVID-19-related murder-suicide by gunshot. Mr. Jesernik shot his partner (who had been suffering from severe breathing problems) before killing himself. He was scared that he had been infected with COVID-19 from his girlfriend. Both had been tested for COVID-19 but it appears neither had received their results before their deaths. The autopsies showed that neither was infected with COVID-19.

An Indian elderly couple from Amritsar, India – Balwinder Singh (aged 65) and his wife Gurinder Kaur (age not reported) – committed suicide by consuming a poisonous substance together. Their suicide note said there was tension because of COVID-19. Their suicide note simply said: 'We are finishing our lives. No one is responsible for this. There has been a tension due to coronavirus. We both were also ill.' The police reported they were not actually infected with COVID-19.

A young newlywed couple from Uttarakhand, India – Ashok Kumar (aged 24) and his wife Rajju Devi (age not reported) – both committed suicide together by hanging themselves from a tree.

Mr. Kumar had been quarantined (after returning from Punjab) at a school that had been turned into an isolation centre near his village. Although he had no COVID-19 symptoms, he was prevented from going home and his wife was being pressured and harassed by neighbours to leave the village because they all thought Mr. Kumar had COVID-19. The wife visited her husband at the quarantine centre and both felt the situation was hopeless so committed suicide together in a forest nearby the centre.

A man from Bihar, India – Ramesh Shah (aged 35) – committed suicide by hanging himself after his wife (Suman, age not reported) committed suicide by setting herself on fire. The couple were unable to pay back a loan on a truck they had bought because they were unable to work during the COVID-19 lockdown. After an argument concerning their finances, Suman deliberately set herself on fire. The husband tried to save his wife but she died at hospital. The husband was so distraught that he then killed himself. The couple left behind two young children (aged 7 and 10).

Dr Richard Seiden[7] has investigated those who have been bodily restrained from leaping to their deaths off the Golden Gate bridge by the California Highway Patrol or workers on the bridge. He tracked down 515 people who had attempted to jump off the bridge over thirty-five years, finding at the time of his study that 94 per cent either were still alive or had died of natural causes, and only 6 per cent had committed suicide or died in accidents suggestive of suicide. It would seem that once you make the effort to prevent self-destruction, the vast majority of potential victims recover from their prior state of hopelessness and despair.

Paradoxically enough, there is another, more hopeful possible ending to this story of suicide.

In his book *November of the Soul – The Enigma of Suicide*, George Howe Colt[8] reports the following astonishing true story.

When a suicidal eighteen-year-old girl balanced precariously on the edge of a towering seven-storey building in Mexico City, apparently about to leap, Ignacio Canedo, an eighteen-year-old Red Cross nurse, carefully, slowly, sidled out to her. Canedo was secured to a stretched line, gripped on the other end by a crew of firemen.

'Don't come any nearer!' the girl screamed in warning. 'Don't or I'll jump!' Canedo lunged for her but grasped empty air. The girl shrieked and sprang. He dived after her and seized her mid-plummet, his arms encircling her waist. They tumbled fiour floors before the rope whipped and cracked tight. Canedo's grip held. He and the sobbing girl were dragged back to the roof.

'I knew the rope would save me,' said Canedo. 'I prayed that it would be strong enough to support both of us.'

Behind all the depressing suicide statistics, how many dozens, if not hundreds, of similar tales are there that we never hear of? Certain deaths prevented by strangers who just intuitively reached out?[9]

5

DON'T CRY FOR ME, CORONA

Is crying good for you?

On the morning of Tuesday, 8 December 2020, Matt Hancock, the UK Minister for Health, appeared tearful during live TV footage of the first man in the UK to receive the anti-coronavirus vaccine.

A normally cynical press appeared to be similarly moved; the headline in the *Daily Express* read, 'MATT HANCOCK broke down in tears on Tuesday's edition of *Good Morning Britain* as the first-ever coronavirus vaccine in the world had been administered in the UK,' while the normally hard-nosed presenter Piers Morgan declared that the politician was 'visibly moved'.

But is there something cheeky going on here? *The Guardian* maintained that the Conservative minister's face remained stubbornly dry; the tears looked fake to them.

One way of thinking about crying is that there are different types of tears. One sort reveals inner turmoil, while another might represent a collision with the outside world.

In the midst of the pandemic, the crying certainly seems contagious amongst politicians: Angela Merkel's voice 'cracked' in the same week while passionately urging adherence to Germany's latest coronavirus rules.

Observers report feeling more connected to people who are crying, and this powerfully enhances the willingness of bystanders to help the tearful. If tears signal helplessness, then are our leaders resorting to wailing in an attempt to emotionally blackmail us into lockdown, or vaccine, obedience?

A team of researchers[1] from the University of València in Spain, showed the public photographs of tearful people, and also a control group of the same pictures with the tears digitally removed, together with brief descriptions of crimes supposedly committed by the photographed.

The study found that crying made those who appeared to have committed criminal acts appear more sincere, reliable, kind and remorseful. Depending on how closely you feel politicians resemble criminals, it might be the findings help explain Matt Hancock's crying.

But while the convicted person was viewed as kinder, more honest, and more remorseful when presented with tears than without tears, this didn't have such a powerful effect when it came to the public deciding over handing down punishment for these crimes. Tears only affected the severity of the proposed punishment in the specific case of drink-driving, where shorter sentences were proposed for tearful perpetrators (irrespective of gender) than for their tearless counterparts.

Maybe the public is alive to the possibly manipulative aspect of crying. Humans may be unique amongst animals in shedding tears for purely emotional reasons; sincerity may be more of an issue between people than it is between animals.

But is sobbing actually good for you? Does it relieve stress? Does it depend on the kind of tears and the circumstances?

If crying becomes helpful because of the sympathetic and supportive emotional reaction it provokes in others, does weeping alone become counterproductive, as it doesn't galvanise others to offer support when in fact that is the whole point of crying?

On 28 December 2020, BBC News[2] reported that Dr Bethan Gibson, a senior intensive care doctor at the Royal Glamorgan Hospital, admitted to having cried more during the pandemic than over the span of her entire career. Clinicians, particularly those staffing intensive care units, were especially stressed.

Normally patients on intensive care units are too ill to be that conscious of their situation, but those suffering from COVID-19 were often awake and aware on the ward, despite being very sick. What particularly upset Dr Gibson was witnessing the 'fear in the eyes' of patients being told they may not survive the illness: '… now acutely aware of how sick there are, they're begging and pleading with us to make sure they don't die,' she said.

Was crying so much helping this senior doctor deal with her predicament, or might it possibly be a sign she was not coping so well at times?

BBC Radio 3, with a reputation for being the radio channel for the super-refined and ultra-intelligent, launched a series entitled 'Tearjerker', which was its attempt to provide what *The Daily Telegraph*'s music critic described as an 'aural comfort blanket' during the pandemic.

The station explained that Tearjerker[3] 'encourages listeners to press play and shed a tear, exploring the healing powers of sad music, from piano classics such as [the] Moonlight Sonata by Beethoven to the soothing electronica of artists like James Blake'.

Does the psychological research support the idea that a good cry alone with the radio represents 'healing', or could it in fact undermine the process?

Psychologists Asmir Gračanin, Lauren Bylsma and Ad Vingerhoets[4] argue in their study entitled 'Why Only Humans Shed Emotional Tears – Evolutionary and Cultural Perspectives' that weeping galvanises support and help from others, partly because it's potentially a strong signal of genuine despair.

The roots of crying may lie in the fact babies cry a lot, because human infants are unique amongst animals in being so helpless and powerless over such an extended period, during which they are particularly vulnerable if abandoned by their caregivers.[5] Unlike other primates, they cannot cling to their mother's fur, while movement remains so undeveloped for so long that they can't independently motor after their mothers for years – unlike, for example, the offspring of geese and ducks.[4]

It is therefore no accident, according to these psychologists, that human infants initiate crying when set down and stop when scooped up. Babies hardly ever cry when carried in a sling, which produces continuous physical contact with mum. Weeping becomes an essential 'acoustic umbilical cord', maintaining proximity between baby and parent.[4]

But even babies may already be crying for manipulative reasons. Bawling evolved generations ago when our ancestral environment was teeming with predators, so parents would have been motivated to pay attention urgently, and soothe a crying newborn fast, in order to prevent unwanted attention from enemies prowling the undergrowth.[5]

A vigorously weeping baby may occupy the attention of parents so much that it precludes them procreating again, so a crying baby may be in fact be scheming to reduce potential sibling competition.[4]

If we have evolved more complex facial musculature than other animals, partly to suckle milk and to communicate emotions through facial expression, then why then did we need tears on top of an upset face or screaming bellow?[4] Tears draw attention to the eyes, and are difficult to make out from far away, so crying might be designed as a specific signal for those particularly close to us.[5]

The debate over whether Matt Hancock had really cried or not partly occurred because no one was that near to him at the time. We are uncomfortable making too much eye contact with strangers, but it is required in intimate relationships.

An international study[6] by psychologist Ad Vingerhoets, with more than 5,500 adult participants, has established that the most common time to shed tears is between 7.00 p.m. and 10.00 p.m. This is when we are most likely to be alone with intimates, hence the increased likelihood of arguments with those to whom we are closest. The absence of strangers who might otherwise inhibit crying, plus the fact it's toward the end of the day when we are more tired, may also be relevant.[7]

If crying is about intimate connection, then what is going on when people cry in public or at work? As in the case of Matt Hancock?

Kimberly Elsbach and Beth Bechky[8] published a study which evaluated female colleagues who teared up in the office. If the female professionals were guilty of breaking the rules of their job, and this explained why they were sobbing, observers tended to conclude they were weak, unprofessional and manipulative. If, however, they were not guilty of any violations, then criers were perceived more positively, as experiencing a tough situation at work, or personal issues at home.

At the extreme end of professional tears are the professional criers or wailers prevalent in some non-Western cultures,[9] mourners who appear at funerals, for example. Their presence appears specifically designed to help others cry, as a cathartic and healing process. Sobbing together may serve a particularly unique bonding experience, which we in the West look down on as excessive public emotionality.

But people don't just lament at funerals, they also weep at weddings, in very positive situations, such as witnessing the intensification of relationships, or extraordinary generosity, selflessness or exceptional performances. Crying may signal a shared value system at these exclamation-mark moments. Are we mourning or celebrating the rarity of the special commitment being demonstrated? Or both?

Gračanin, Bylsma and Vingerhoets point out in their study that there is a remarkable custom among a substantial number of South American Indian tribes, but also in North America, Australia, India, and the

Andaman Islands, where peoples greet arriving strangers while shedding copious tears. Michael Harbsmeier,[10] an anthropologist and historian, reports on the phenomenon in his study entitled 'Why do the Indians cry?':

> The traveller is first led to the hut where he is to live; the women gather around the hammock in which the traveller has been laid, cover their faces with their hands and give themselves up to a quite appalling fit of weeping … the crying women then lament not only all the death and tragedies that have befallen them and their village, but also the many dangers and accidents that the traveller himself has undergone in order to reach his destination. After a while, this ceremonial crying and lamenting stops again, and the traveller can get up from his hammock and give his own account of his experiences to those gathered.

This ceremonial and ritual sharing of tears comes from more ancient cultures used to surviving disaster more frequently than we in the pampered West ever had to. Does the pandemic mean we should develop in response new, similar ceremonies and rituals to share and expunge grief?

In the UK there were national group sharing events like 'clap for carers' but there was never going to be a 'cry for carers' or equivalent, as that would have been out of keeping with our culture. Though sometimes despite ourselves tears were shed. The last time we as a nation collectively really cried was following the death of Princess Diana. What does it say about how the media and officialdom handled the pandemic, that we appeared more united in grief back then than we do now?

As we all took precautions to insulate against the virus, did we experience the painful defencelessness of the more helpless, or did we protect ourselves from sharing this emotional pain? Did we shed a tear only for those close to us and not for any strangers, unlike these supposedly more 'primitive' tribes?

Did you 'buy' Health Minister Matt Hancock's own explanation for his tears which arrived as he watched someone remotely on a TV screen receive a jab – 'It's just been such a tough year for so many people' – yet none of whom he may have known personally?

Maybe when people cry, how they weep reveals more about their psychology than the actual tears themselves.

In 2012 Andy Murray lost the Wimbledon final to Roger Federer, and bravely fought back tears as he attempted to congratulate the Swiss 'time machine' on winning. It seemed to summarise poignantly an important shift in the British psyche from the days of Empire and 'stiff upper lip'. The North Americans and Australians, both sport- and winning-obsessed cultures, remain perplexed as to how the British now love a weeping loser, it appears, more than a winner. The nation as a whole warmed to Andy Murray, it would seem, more than if he had won.

This was back in 2012, and Murray commented in his speech on how the thirty-year-old Federer, astonishingly, had enormous fight left in him despite his age. Who would have guessed that eight years later, Roger Federer would still be up there, competing against the best?

Which elite athlete's reaction helps us most to understand resilience in the face of enormous adversity? Could you predict the divergence in careers from this emotional moment? The highly charged spectacle raised a major question: does our emotional reaction reveal our resilience? Might this dramatic weeping predict future performance in similar high-stress situations?

A sea of tears will have been wept before the pandemic is over, but is crying good for you?

The latest psychological research on whether crying is useful for us suggests that the media consensus on Murray's tears being fine (see how the nation warmed to him) may be missing an important point.

There are *different kinds of crying* and the reason you are sobbing determines whether you benefit from a good weep or not.

There are contrasting types of tears, just as there are distinct versions of happiness. In a book entitled *Men Don't Cry, Women Do: Transcending Gender Stereotypes of Grief*[11] by Terry Martin and Kenneth Doka, a thesis is advanced that there are two main ways of grieving. 'Instrumental grievers' are 'cognitive' and 'active'. They are trying to learn why they are feeling rotten and endeavouring to do something about it – like the bereaved constructing a memorial. The other main style of grieving, referred to as 'intuitive', the authors argue, is more 'feminine' – it involves expressing strong emotion which pulls in support.

In a study entitled 'Culture and Crying: Prevalences and Gender Differences',[12] it is reported that Darwin found that in England and the West generally, crying was less common than in non-Western cultures. This same paper also reports that the first cross-cultural study, published in 1906, concluded that 'tears are more frequently shed among the lower races of mankind than among civilized people'.

To re-investigate this claim, redolent with the arrogant racism of its era, using modern data, the paper conducted a cross-cultural study of adult crying across thirty-seven countries. Men in Malaysia come out as least likely to cry across the world while Italian men are found to have the highest tendency to weep worldwide. In terms of Andy Murray and Roger Federer, yes, the study found men in the UK are more likely to cry than those in Switzerland.

The study also revealed that men and women living in wealthier, democratic, extraverted and individualistic nations, report crying more often. The authors of the study conclude that weeping across the world relates more to freedom of expression than to actual suffering. They argue this explains why the tendency to cry is found to be larger in societies that score higher in subjective well-being.

In a study entitled 'When is crying cathartic? An international study',[6] psychologists found that crying is not necessarily always so good for us.

When asked to recall their last episode of weeping, most participants in the study reported feeling better afterwards; it seems at first glance that crying must be a good thing – the release of assumed tension means we generally feel psychologically improved afterwards. This fits with another curious finding from previous research, which is that more severely clinically depressed patients often seem, paradoxically, less able to cry.

But analysing the latest data more deeply should lead us to wonder if crying is always beneficial, and therefore whether Murray's outburst is in fact good for him in the longer term.

The authors point out that studies exposing subjects to sad movies found mostly a negative effect of shedding tears: those who cried while watching a sad film tended to be more depressed afterwards compared to those who did not cry. When we get upset our physiology is profoundly affected. Yet the mixed findings of these academic studies mean that the jury is still out on whether heart rate and blood pressure recover more rapidly after a crying spell: which is surprising, if crying was indeed so good for you.

Perhaps the rather cold, indifferent atmosphere of a laboratory means that crying doesn't get a chance to perform as powerfully as it does in real life. After all, nothing binds us together or makes others more sympathetic and helpful to us than the natural human response to tears.

Criticism of Andy Murray's performance during the aforementioned match has been almost completely deflected by his crying, which demonstrates the true clout of tears. What other force on the planet could produce such a total media somersault in coverage of this character, viewed before as truculent and aloof, by the unforgiving press?

To get more definitively to the bottom of crying, one of the largest studies on sobbing by Bylsma, Rottenberg and colleagues,[7] asked ninety-seven female students with an average age of twenty to keep a 'crying and mood diary' for approximately two months.

The study, entitled, 'When and for whom does crying improve mood?', using a daily diary study of 1,004 crying episodes, found that in two months the average young woman cries ten times. Prior research had found the equivalent number for men to be around two times over the same period.

The study reports an average duration of crying of eight minutes, and that these episodes were most often in the living room (40.1 per cent) or bedroom (28.6 per cent). Most were either alone (37.9 per cent) or with one other person (39.8 per cent). The most common reasons for crying were conflict (16.3 per cent), loss (13.5 per cent) or witnessing the suffering of others (13.1 per cent).

A principal finding of the study with particular relevance to any elite athlete,[13] for whom emotional control is going to be vital in predicting future success, is that those who are more prone to cry also suffer more mood variability. The study found emotionally laden tears were followed by a period of worsened mood, with no apparent benefit.

In other words, crying was *not* seen by these researchers as generally good for us.

However, 30 per cent of crying episodes – a distinct minority – were associated with mood improvement and these seemed to be when weeping occurred with greater *intensity* (but not duration). Perhaps more intense crying may be more likely to attract social support – an echo of the Andy Murray incident?

The authors conclude that, generally, crying is not good for us, except for those specific moments when others around us – because they are close to us – are going to be positively supportive and responsive to our tears. If we experience a resolution to the difficult circumstances that caused the crying episode – perhaps because of the new sympathy of others, or because we achieve a new more positive understanding of the predicament through our tears – then in these special circumstances, crying is good for us. Expressing grief does sometimes lead us to a different and better understanding of ourselves.

Crying appears to be particularly unhelpful if we cry in the presence of others who are unsympathetic. But in Murray's case it appears to have rallied the nation, which might have proven useful in future on-court battles.

We cry when we are unable to solve a serious problem that we are facing. Tears represent an energy that would be better used in acting on a solution, and crying appears particularly unhelpful where we have little control over the upsetting incident, such as witnessing suffering or conflict.

Andy may have solved one crisis by crying – he galvanised a nation to support him. But crying would not have helped with the other emergencies he so bravely faced on the tennis court. The tears might be a sign he was at a complete loss, and alone while in the midst of play.

The suppression of tears in order to fight through and win in the midst of the mental war has been termed 'mental toughness' by sports psychologists. This is a much rarer quality than is commonly realised and in fact probably explains the difference between victory and defeat at the top level of elite sport, even more than technical skill.

But what exactly is 'mental toughness', and how do you get it?

Tim Twietmeyer, who has completed the 100-mile Western States Endurance Run twenty-five times, on each occasion in under twenty-four hours, declared: 'There is nothing noble in being superior to some other man. The true nobility is being superior to your previous self.'[13]

Psychologists agree the toughest challenge that elite athletes face comes not from their opponents, but from themselves.[13]

A basic confusion, however, is to mistake indifference for toughness – the Victorian inhibition of emotions, particularly any sign of vulnerability or weakness – is not the same thing as mental toughness. Mental toughness involves experiencing strong emotions but controlling them.

Tennis star Victoria Azarenka, when she won championship point at the Australian Open in 2013, sobbed dramatically. That intense passion didn't just arrive out of the blue, it was there all along simmering beneath the surface and could have tipped out at any moment given the right ignition.

The dramatic displays of emotion after victory, or defeat, in these champions indicate just how much there is pent up on the inside, and the astonishing level of control being exerted.

There were very different kinds of tears shed by the same Azarenka on 16 January 2019 when she broke down during a press conference following her first-round loss at the Australian Open. She has had off-court battles to fight: injuries, and custody cases over her child. She may be much more robust in one kind of court than another, showing that resilience is something you have to train for.

Similarly, anyone who saw Novak Djokovic pound his racket into submission on the court floor in his early days would not view him as 'unemotional'.

The mentally tough self-regulate, controlling impulses and emotions. They have superior self-confidence, appraisal of achievements, self-esteem, sense of purpose and contribution, self-efficacy, belief in abilities and strengths, and also self-control. The belief that one is in control of one's life is paramount: captain of your ship and master of your fate.

No matter how much support any tennis player has from those close to them, their fans and even the entire country, tennis remains the loneliest game. Andre Agassi once said:

> Only boxers can understand the loneliness of tennis players – and
> yet boxers have their corner men and managers … The rules forbid
> a tennis player from even talking to [the] coach while on the court.

We cry when we feel sorry for ourselves. Tears reveal inner turmoil. We weep in victory and in defeat. Because it's about a loss of control we can fail to see, even at this of all moments, that's it's vital to consider what ultimate purpose howling, bawling or whimpering serves.

As some suggest, in tennis, as in life, the only person we ever really lose against is ourselves.

6

HOW COVID KILLED COMEDY: DOES HUMOUR REALLY HELP HEAL?

It's a pundemic

There is controversy as to whether Sigmund Freud ever actually told this joke[1] (he did write the least funny book ever published, 'Jokes and their relation to the Unconscious'), but for the sake of understanding the psychology behind humour, lets 'just go with it', to borrow a phrase from a recent Adam Sandler rom-com.

The founder of psychoanalysis sailed for the USA from Europe on 21 August 1909, with his travelling companions including perhaps the second most famous therapist of all time, Carl Gustav Jung. Freud had been invited to give a series of lectures at Clark University, Massachusetts, so this was a crossroads moment in the history of psychotherapy. Following his talks, psychoanalysis spread like a raging epidemic across the USA, soon becoming the most popular treatment for mental illness in the country.

As their liner cruised through the mouth of the Hudson, on the evening of 29 August 1909, gripped by the startling skyline of the New World, Freud, it is sometimes claimed, turned to Jung and uttered these words: 'They don't realize that we're bringing them the plague.' 'The plague' in this instance is supposed to be a reference to the idea Freud was carrying psychoanalysis, a revolutionary new treatment, to North America from Europe, but which was so controversial, it could be regarded more as a disease than a panacea.

Later Carl Gustav Jung reported that what Freud actually said was, 'If they only knew what we are bringing to them.'

The first version is a kind of joke, but with such a lot going on beneath the surface, it could not just entertain but also transform the way the listener thinks. Is this humour as a real impactful mental treatment, as opposed to jokes as a sort of quick chemical hit?

Jokes can cheer you up momentarily, and maybe that is enough, given the desperate need for stress relief in a time of plague.

But is that all humour can achieve? Or can deeper, more insightful wit help us cope by working at a more fundamental level on our psychology? Can some sense of humour even be counter-productive in terms of mental health? How to tell the difference? Here are some pandemic jokes widely circulating on the internet.[2]

> Nothing like relaxing on the couch after a long day of being tense on the couch.
>
> I'm just a boy, standing six feet away from a girl. Asking you to maybe move back another foot. Thanks.
>
> 30 days hath September, April, June, and November, all the rest have 31, except for March which was infinite.
>
> I finished Netflix today.
>
> Day 121 at home and the dog is looking at me like, 'See? This is why I chew the furniture.'

By the end of this chapter you should be able to work out which of the witticisms above would score higher on helping you cope with the pandemic in a deeper sense than just bringing a smile, or laugh, and therefore merely momentary reprieve.

Stand-up comedians who ply their trade with funny observations about life have struggled to make jokes about COVID-19. Paradoxically, in contrast, the internet has been awash with amusing video clips and memes composed by the public deploying humour as a coping skill, helping them deal with the pandemic.

Why the strange gap in productivity between the amateurs and the professionals? Particularly just when everyone was looking for something funny to take their mind off things?

This may partly be because the industry, as with much live performance, has itself has been decimated by the virus. Comedians thrown out of work are having to take up other occupations to make ends meet. They have become very worried about whether they or even the whole business has a future. The key word here is business; it may be a different enterprise when humour is your livelihood, as opposed to your hobby.

Stand-up comedy also employs a host of other professions, not just agents but front-of-house staff and bartenders, all of whom have found themselves out of work with their prospects extremely precarious. Maybe if you are on the inside or close to all that misery, it's difficult to make fun of the predicament.

In addition, some famous comedians have themselves been killed by COVID-19 including Tim Brook-Taylor and Eddie Large, real name Edward McGinnis, part of the comedy double act Little and Large. The conceit of the double act was that Syd Little, the 'straight' man in the double act, would look bemused and even alarmed at various strange impressions that the 'funny' man, Eddie Large, would introduce. Yet there is some scientific research from before the virus came along which predicts with amazing accuracy which member of a comedy double-act is more likely to die first.

The research draws attention to the deeper question of where a sense of humour comes from. Does the source link to deeper aspects of our personality which can predict our longevity?

Is this evidence a sign that the virus represents a difficulty too far, so even humour can't help us cope? A seductive idea at first glance, that you could laugh your way out of trouble, but there are serious problems with this approach.

Not least is the fact that those who are supposed to have the best sense of humour of all, comedians, appear to suffer from high rates of depression and even suicide. If humour is a good coping strategy, how to explain the reputed adverse link between professional humorists and mental health?

For example, in August 2014, aged sixty-three, the talented comedian and very funny actor Robin Williams committed suicide by hanging at his home in Paradise Cay, California. The autopsy did attribute his suicide to struggles with Lewy body disease, a form of dementia. But the star's publicist, Mara Buxbaum, also said Williams had recently been suffering from severe depression. The tragedy might be explained by some psychologists' argument that this is because many comedians appear somewhat 'manic-depressive'.

Along with a team of researchers, Victoria Ando from St Hugh's College, University of Oxford, has published a study entitled 'Psychotic Traits in Comedians',[3] which uncovers a link between the manic side of bipolar disorder and comic performance. The research argues for links between mania and comedy through very high mood, combining with rapidly changing ideas.

The study points to the notable example of famous English comedian Spike Milligan, who experienced manic-depressive episodes throughout his life.

The researchers argue that Milligan used the freely associating thought processes of his manic states to generate the zany ideas that were the hallmark of his jesting. The same could possibly be posited about Robin Williams.

The study argues for another possible link between being a professional comedian and despair, which is that depression might motivate a talented humorist to find ways of alleviating the low mood. Joking becomes a form of self-medication.

The authors quote poet and writer Antonin Artaud, who himself experienced serious mental illness, writing, 'No one has ever written, painted or sculpted, modelled, built or invented except literally to get out of hell.'

The study compared 523 comedians with 364 actors, and found comics behaved like other creative groups in showing high levels of psychotic personality traits. The most striking result, however, was the comedians' unusual personality profile, featuring 'introverted anhedonia' (anhedonia refers to an inability to take any pleasure from life) and 'extraverted impulsiveness'. This combines seemingly opposite personality characteristics: unsociable, depressive traits and more extraverted, manic-like features.

Intriguingly, female comics scored even higher than male comedians on 'Impulsive Non-conformity' – a tendency towards impulsive, antisocial behaviour, often suggesting a lack of self-control linked to moods. One speculation is perhaps female comics have to be more extreme on these traits in the first place in order to break into the profession.

The authors of the study conclude that this profile of a comedian represents the personality equivalent of bipolar disorder.

Victoria Ando and colleagues point out that humorist Stephen Fry, diagnosed with bipolar disorder, confessed to a suicide bid, and has explained the link with his sense of humour. They quote Fry as referring to his role as the jokey compere of the humorous quiz show *QI*: 'There are times when I'm doing QI and I'm going "ha ha, yeah, yeah", and inside I'm going "I want to fucking die. I ... want ... to ... fucking ... die."'

Fry's comment, the authors argue, illustrates how two conflicting emotional traits typically found in comics might be aroused concurrently, one being used to cope with the other. Psychoanalysts refer to this as the 'manic defence'.

But if humour is supposed to defend against low mood – when doesn't it work? Why does the depression sometimes break through the manic defence, occasionally leading to suicide? Suicidal levels of depression have been linked to many successful comedians, including Tony Hancock and Kenneth Williams.

One possible answer comes from psychological research which suggests the secret might lie in the style of humour you adopt as your way of coping with life's adversities.[4]

The study, entitled 'The moderating effect of humor style on the relationship between interpersonal predictors of suicide and suicidal ideation', investigated the psychological impact of two positive (affiliative and self-enhancing) and two negative (aggressive and self-defeating) styles of humour. The study looked at whether it's possible to distinguish different senses of humour people tend to use, and whether this can be revealing of your personality.

An 'affiliative' humour style refers to a tendency to facilitate relationships, reducing interpersonal stress with playful teasing. 'Self-enhancing' humour involves having a humorous outlook on life, especially during stressful times. 'Aggressive' humour refers to disparagement used to manipulate others, such as sarcasm, ridicule, and hostile teasing. Self-defeating humour involves amusing others by doing or saying comical things at one's own expense.

The authors found those who naturally use self-defeating humour are at more of a risk for suicidal thinking when experiencing common stresses, such as feelings of 'thwarted belongingness' or 'perceived burdensomeness'.

'Thwarted belongingness' is a feeling of absence of connectedness to those closest, and a lack of caring from others. 'Perceived burdensomeness' means just what it says, the belief that one is a burden on others. Both 'thwarted belongingness' and 'perceived burdensomeness' have been found to be important in explaining how suicidal people feel.

The study found that it was the 'affiliative' humour style which was particularly protective against feeling suicidal. Of all four humour styles, only 'affiliative' protected significantly against suicidal feelings. Affiliative humour might even defend against depression.

The authors conclude that their results indicate that the ability to use affiliative humour to strengthen interpersonal connections and ease social tensions may be particularly protective against thoughts of suicide.

Humour may serve as either a buffer or a risk factor for suicide – it depends on the kind of comedy deployed. Affiliative humour seems to serve as a buffer, while self-defeating jokes reveal a more negative coping style, exacerbating feelings of loneliness and burdensomeness.

This study suggests that clinicians treating depression might even in future consider monitoring the sense of humour being deployed by their patients as indicating risk of suicide.

The authors argue that those who use self-defeating humour may also be more likely to feel socially disconnected and burdensome to others. Their flaws are constantly being confirmed, through hilarity, by the reactions of others.

Interestingly, although this study was conducted long before the lockdown and the pandemic, it appears to have a direct link with coping strategy during this time of social distancing and isolation. It's suggesting that the right kind of wit, not just a sense of humour, might be helpful because it might promote social connectedness, while the wrong kind could pander to feelings of being aggrieved and exacerbate isolation.

Comedy is clearly a deep and powerful force in the world, as exemplified by another recent intriguing study mentioned earlier, which found that it was possible to predict which half of a comedy duo would live the longest, and that this prediction might even reveal something about the psychology of longevity.

The newspapers are seemingly always reporting the death of one half of a comedy duo long before or after the demise of their partner. For example, the death of Ronnie Corbett, one of Britain's most popular and loved TV comedians, was announced in 2016 – he was eighty-five. Corbett was possibly best known as one half of a comedy duo referred to as 'The Two Ronnies', a popular British TV series boasting a comedy partner, Ronnie Barker, who died in 2005, aged seventy-six. The study,[5] recently published in the *International Journal of Cardiology*, found that the funniest comedians suffer dramatically reduced longevity, compared to their relatively less funny counterparts.

The research analysed the life span of fifty-three male British comedians born between 1900 and 1954. The higher the score by which the comedian was rated as funny, the higher the mortality rate. Of the twenty-three 'very funny' comedians, 78 per cent had died, versus 40 per cent of the rest. Average age at death for the comedians adjudged as 'very funny' was 63.3 years, compared with 72.3 for the rest.

Those working in comedy duos (e.g. Morecambe and Wise) or teams (e.g. Monty Python) were also designated, for the purposes of this research, as the 'funny' or 'straight' men in that comedy team. Within comedy teams, those identified as the funnier member(s) of the partnership were more than three times more likely to die prematurely when compared to their more serious comedy partners.

Examples that bear out that the funny man in a comedy team seems to always die first include Ernie Wise being the straighter comedian in the duo, living to seventy-three, while his more overtly funny partner, Eric Morecambe, died at fifty-eight. Ronnie Barker died at seventy-six while his straight man Ronnie Corbett was eighty-five. Not much in it. However, there might be come controversy as to whether Corbett really was the straight man to Barker in this particular duo.

Graham Chapman died at forty-eight, while most of the other original members of the Monty Python comedy team – John Cleese, Eric Idle, Michael Palin, Terry Gilliam (but sadly not Terry Jones who died in January 2020) – are still alive at the time of writing. It is widely argued that Chapman was the most surreal, or the funniest, of this uniquely surreal comedy team. For example, perhaps the most famous Monty Python sketch of all, the 'Dead Parrot' sketch, was written by John Cleese as about a man returning a toaster, yet it is sometimes suggested that it was Chapman who inspired the idea it should be about a dead parrot.

The findings of this study[5] are particularly intriguing because, consistent with the inherent nature of comedy tandems and teams, individual members were predominantly born around the same time, and come from the same social class and economic background. The authors conclude that elite comedians are at increased risk of premature death, compared to their less funny counterparts.

The study involved ranking all fifty-three comedians according to their ability to make people laugh on a numbered scale. Some scored as 'relatively funny', others scoring higher were found 'pretty funny' and the best were rated 'very funny' to 'hilarious'. This last group would be considered 'elite' comedians and include John Cleese and Billy Connolly.

The study used a popular website that ranks the best of only British and Irish comedians. The researchers therefore focused on a group of comedians from only one geographical part of the world. But the authors argue that a preliminary examination of the comedy scene outside of the

UK suggests that their study reveals a more universal phenomenon. For example, the survival profiles of famous and celebrated comedy duos such as Abbott ('funny' partner who died aged fifty-two) and Costello (straight man who died aged seventy-eight) suggest these findings may hold true across the Atlantic and elsewhere.

The authors point out that previous research has established that comedians score high on measures of psychotic traits, and display an unusual personality structure characterised by that 'introverted anhedonia' (an inability to find pleasure in normally pleasurable activities) combined with 'extraverted impulsiveness'.

One theory is that there is something about the kind of personality and psychology involved in being particularly funny linked to this high mortality rate. The authors of the study point out that many comedians have publicly admitted to being depressed, or manic, or sometimes even both. Examples include John Cleese, Peter Cook, Stephen Fry, Tony Hancock, Spike Milligan and Kenneth Williams. In the case of some like Tony Hancock (widely regarded as a comic genius), this resulted in his taking his own life. The study was partly inspired by the suicide of comedian Robin Williams.

Suicide alone cannot, however, account for this finding, as many of the comedians who died early did so from natural or medical causes, not suicide, including the recent death, aged just fifty-six, of funnyman Rik Mayall, reportedly from a heart attack. It may be such personalities manifest self-destructiveness in some more long-term ways and don't look after themselves – although it is reported that Graham Chapman eventually managed to give up alcohol, it is also rumoured that he took up drinking as a medical student to cover his shyness.

Psychologists compared the personalities of thirty-one professional stand-up comedians with those of nine amateur comedians, ten humour writers and 400 college students. 'The Big Five personality traits of professional comedians compared to amateur comedians, comedy writers, and college students'[6] found that, surprisingly, comedians are more introverted than other people.

The authors argue that you would expect comedians' pursuit of fame and attention to mean they are bound to be highly extravert, as we know actors tend to be. The intriguing result suggests that comedians do not seek fame in the same way as actors do.

While the authors of the study acknowledge that the public perceive comedians as ostentatious and flashy, perhaps their persona on stage is mistakenly seen as interchangeable with their real personality. The jokes they tell about their lives might be considered by many to contain a grain of truth in them; however, the results of this study suggest that the opposite is true.

The authors speculate that perhaps comedians use their performance to disguise who they are in their daily life. Comedians may portray someone they want to be, or perhaps their act is a way of defying the constraints imposed on their everyday events and interactions with others.

The authors contend that 'impulsive dis-inhibition' is at the core of the comedic personality, and is necessary to constantly come up with weird new ideas that are funny. Comedians also need this to violate social rules by publicly declaring unconventional sentiments. But does this 'impulsive dis-inhibition' end up killing them, because they then don't look after themselves properly?

If a sense of humour is helping you connect with others, therefore staving off social isolation during a pandemic, or is assisting you in distracting yourself from stressful predicaments, then this is all to the good. However, beware: a sense of humour taken too far appears to be linked with not looking after yourself properly, and this is absolutely vital during a pandemic.

Those who bring the house down also seem to pull the curtain down too quickly.

Katie Watson published an academic study entitled 'Gallows Humour in Medicine'[7] about the fact that comedy seems to thrive most in some of the toughest areas of medicine, such as the emergency room or the high-security psychiatric forensic unit – places where, Watson argued, there was little or no hope. She quotes Viktor Frankl, the psychiatrist who survived concentration camps during the Second World War and who was interested in psychological survival in the most brutal and hopeless of circumstances.

Frankl described concentration camp prisoners who still managed to crack jokes about their horrific predicament. For the psychiatrist, 'Humour was another of the soul's weapons in the fight for self-preservation. It is well known that humour, more than anything else in the human make-up, can afford an aloofness and an ability to rise above any situation, even if only for a few seconds.'

Katie Watson contends that humour plays a vital psychological role in keeping a person engaged in a situation where suicide might seem to be the only real option. She quotes writer George Saunders: 'Humour is what happens when we're told the truth quicker and more directly than we're used to.'

But this refers to sophisticated comedy, which seeks to do more than just entertain or divert. With truly great comedy, we laugh because the joke reveals some deep insight. There is a confrontation with an uncomfortable truth, but by facing it we also at that very moment become more powerful because we stop running away.

Katie Watson quotes a joke based on a true story told to her by an emergency department physician. I don't want to spell out in too much detail the analogy with what the virus is doing to us, but here goes the true story:

> A thief escaping from a bank robbery crashed his car, and the police brought him to the emergency room for a trauma evaluation on his way to jail. That includes a rectal exam, and the emergency room doctor expected the prisoner to object, as many of the big tough guys he treats do. Instead, when the doctor asked, 'I need to do a rectal exam,' the prisoner looked out at the sea of cops and said, 'I guess I have to get used to it.'

And one final joke, which is in a sense the pandemic joke to end all pandemic jokes, because it sobers up to make us re-think our future. It comes from Alfred Crosby's book,[8] *America's Forgotten Pandemic: The Influenza of 1918* and is quoted in Elizabeth Rottenberg's study 'Theory in a Time of Plague':

> There is a bitter little pill of a joke currently circulating among infectious disease experts. It is short: the nineteenth century was followed by the twentieth century, which was followed by the ... nineteenth century.

7

DOES COVID ALSO KILL BY BORING YOU TO DEATH?

Could the boredom be more dangerous than the virus?

Pope Francis has an official Instagram account[1] which, somewhat unexpectedly, recently 'liked' a photograph of a Brazilian bikini model sporting a skimpy 'schoolgirl' outfit, including a very short mini skirt, suspenders and stockings. Twenty-seven-year-old Ms Natalia Garibotto is pictured posing provocatively in front of a school locker. Her fingers have closed over a book in the locker, as she looks back, provocatively, over her shoulder at you. The caption beneath the picture reads, 'I can teach you a thing or two.' Pope Francis is highly active on social media, with 7.4 million followers.

Press speculation is that someone in the Holy See's communications team must have accidentally (an act of God?) pressed the 'like' button, while perusing the model's vast gallery of risqué images. Ms Garibo has responded to the furore by declaring the 'like' means, she insists, 'At least I'm going to heaven.' The fact the 'like' was removed a day later, I hope, doesn't mean her eventual destination has now changed. She joked in the midst of the furore, 'Be right back, on my way to the Vatican.'

When we get bored, we can end up indulging in some rather aberrant, perhaps even incomprehensible actions. Listlessness might in part account for the Dominic Cummings and Neil Ferguson debacles. Tedium turns juveniles into delinquents, and maybe even transforms adults into juveniles. This powerful dreariness effect of the pandemic's restrictions on activities could even explain how delinquency may have broken into no less a moral fortress than the holy Vatican.

Does the fact those closest to God might also get restless tell us just how invidious this is?

If COVID-19 is so serious and tedious that even stand-up comedy finds it no laughing matter, might the monotony of the whole thing also kill us?

As large sections of the world increasingly find themselves restricted in what they are allowed to do, look out for another pandemic – with an even higher infectivity rate than any virus. Boredom is now a serious risk.[2] Could this negative emotional state end up causing more harm that the microbe?

Boredom at first glance seems a common and rather innocuous emotion, but the latest psychological research begs to differ.[3]

Boredom has been blamed for clinical depression, alcoholism, overeating, obesity and drug abuse, and, beyond specialists' clinics, it is considered to be a factor in vandalism and other crimes.[3] It's been linked to gambling, dangerous driving, self-harm and even psychosis.[3]

Interest in boredom has grown recently with a revival of studies into the concept that boredom is a pathological condition. This may explain many current social problems such as youth violence, and other risk-taking behaviour.

Recent studies of school pupils show that while many are bored with at least one subject, a large number find all subjects boring.[4] But it is not just school that these students find boring – they are bored during their spare time as well.

These results suggest that some people may suffer from pathological boredom – not task-linked, but more a characteristic of particular people or their personalities. The same research also suggests that boredom runs in families – bored pupils have bored parents.[3]

It also suggests that boredom decreases with age.[5] People seem most prone to boredom during adolescence.[6] This is when emerging adults are learning to focus their attention in ways that elude younger children. It may be that teenagers who fail to attain an adult ability to concentrate will suffer boredom, and – not ignoring the influence of other factors – turn to crime and drug abuse. The brain-wave patterns characteristic of this 'selective attention' first emerge when a child is about eleven or twelve years old.

The brain's frontal lobes send messages to the rest of the nervous system to inhibit widespread activity, producing concentrated activity in specific areas of the brain.[6] This provides the ability to focus on selective events and so prevents boredom.

Differences in brain activity have been observed, enabling researchers to distinguish between those who are easily distracted and those who can concentrate well.[3]

Boredom is more profound than simply a lack of stimulation. Sometimes it is the lack of any impulse whatsoever. The problem is not finding something to do, it is finding a reason for doing anything at all. This explains the hopeless task of trying to interest some bored people in any subject, despite the most riveting suggestions.[6]

Complaints of feeling bored are common. Surveys have found that 56 per cent of British employees report that they find their entire job boring, while 87 per cent say they feel bored doing their work on some occasions.[3]

Medical research has found that bored workers have three to five times the usual incidence of cardiovascular disease,[6] four to seven times the incidence of neurological disorders, twice the incidence of gastrointestinal disorders and two to three times the incidence of musculo-skeletal disorders.[3]

They are also absent from work for medical reasons three to five times as often as their non-bored colleagues.[6] Swedish research published in 1975 said that 60 per cent of mill workers doing one particularly boring task were receiving treatment for peptic ulcers. Some even complained of hallucinations during periods when they were bored.[3]

This may be explained by the surprising finding that adrenaline levels are twice as high as normal during boring work – in response to frustration. So those with boring jobs experience a great deal of stress.[3] It is possible to be bored to death – literally.[3]

Boredom research is not always predictable; many studies have found industrial workers who claim to enjoy repetitive work. It's not all good, though; a study of female Swiss watchmakers who worked at repetitive tasks found that monotonous jobs lowered the workers' intelligence scores.[3]

Research on long-distance lorry drivers and airline pilots suggests that many motorway pile-ups, air crashes and oil-tanker accidents are directly attributable to boredom. In 1989 the entire cockpit crew of a commercial airline fell asleep and over-flew their destination by more than 100 miles before being awakened by air-traffic controllers, according to a report published in the journal *Human Relations*.[6]

During the Second World War, the RAF was astonished to find that contact with hostile aircraft and U-boats reported by radar operators dropped substantially as more time was spent on duty.[6] Because 50 per cent of targets were being missed, RAF Coastal Command commissioned psychologists to study boredom. Research bodies such as the Industrial Fatigue Research Board had been set up in the 1930s in response to a high level of industrial accidents.[6]

More recent research has identified a sub-type of boredom – 'Sunday boredom'. This is spare-time boredom peculiar to people who succeed in diverting themselves only at work. When distraction is unavailable, latent boredom manifests itself.[6]

Psychopaths – ruthless, self-centred individuals – fall into this group of people who require constant stimulation. They have poor tolerance of routine work and rapidly become blasé about novelty.

Others prone to boredom include those with higher abilities who find most tasks relatively simple, and therefore not as stimulating as they are for the rest of us. Extroverts and the more socially outgoing, surprisingly, suffer more from boredom than introverts. Their high spirits are an attempt to generate the intense levels of stimulation they need to stave off boredom.[6] This subjective experience of time is an important indication of boredom. In an experiment in which psychologists asked people to complete a task in a set time, clocks were tampered with, to run fast or slow. Interest was increased when the clocks were speeded up, and boredom was experienced when they were slowed down. One solution to boredom, then, may be simply allocating less time to boring tasks.[6] In fact, many people already unconsciously do this; they may rush to complete tasks they have put off because they find them boring.

There is a technique called 'distraction management' which identifies occasions or situations in which the subject gets bored and distracted from a task and then removes the distraction.[7] At its most simple level this could mean taking a television set out of the room in which a teenager is doing homework.

Another technique is 'stimulation management', in which the subject is encouraged to use the imagination to keep alert – for example by playing games during a long car drive.[8] This could involve counting Jaguars or red Volkswagens.

One sub-type of boredom was described by an Austrian prince, Field Marshal Charles Joseph de Ligne (1735–1814), a raconteur and socialite who said: 'I am not bored, it is others who bore me.'

Research into what people find boring about each other reveals this is largely based on the quality of conversation. Boring people's conversation was found to be self-centred and trivial while their speech style was slow and low on emotional fervour.

Being boring is a huge social disadvantage – it results in extreme loneliness. As its links with serious personal and social problems become clearer, the need to discover more effective anti-boredom strategies has become more urgent than ever.[7]

Some psychoanalysts believe boredom, if it becomes entrenched, can become a psychiatric disease in itself, and the term 'Alysosis' had been coined to describe such a condition.

Ennui was, historically, something more often associated with the tedium of being at work. Yet what is psychologically novel about the epidemic of monotony now facing us, is that this is the relatively more unusual version of dreariness, termed by psychologists 'leisure boredom'. Because this is a kind of weariness many may not have encountered that much before, they may be much worse at dealing with it.

Severe boredom has been reported in psychiatric academic literature to be linked with a host of psychological problems including paranoia, irritability, aggression and even homicide.

For example, an investigation published in 2018 in the *Journal of Forensic Sciences*[9] into the motivation behind the murder of a sixteen-year-old by two classmates in Idaho, USA, concluded: 'Relief from boredom and the need for fun and excitement, which were evident in the present case, are common motivators to engage in a variety of both legitimate and deviant leisure experiences.' The victim was stabbed thirty times.

Boredom can have fatal consequences, and is also difficult to 'treat'.

The philosopher Friedrich Nietzsche remarked, 'Against boredom even gods struggle in vain.' Fyodor Dostoyevsky, in his novel *Notes from the Underground*, wrote,

Of course boredom may lead you to anything. It is boredom sets one sticking golden pins into people, but all that would not matter. What is bad (this is my comment again) is that I dare say people will be thankful for the gold pins then.

Now the most recent psychological research into boredom has uncovered a tendency for tedium to drive people to more political extremes, as well as encouraging risk-taking and impulsivity.[10]

If these findings are applicable across the world, even when the viral pandemic has subsided we could be left with a much longer-lasting, fundamentally altered political and psychological landscape.

Psychologists Wijnand van Tilburg at the University of Essex and Eric Igou at the University of Limerick, Ireland, published a study entitled 'Going to Political Extremes in Response to Boredom'.[10] They point out that so-called 'existential threat' was previously thought to drive the electorate to embrace political extremes. For example, fanatical politicians induce fear in the electorate by emphasising the danger to society from foreigners and other scapegoats.

The authors contend that those who hold more radical political views have been found to claim a greater sense of understanding of the world, even if their explanations can be overly simplistic or just plain incorrect.[10] The psychology of the predicament when facing threat is that we are driven to look for certainty and coherence.

In which case, one interpretation of this argument is that the current viral pandemic represents a 'double whammy', in terms of pushing the world towards more political extremism. It has created a particularly potent existential threat, perhaps even more alarming to some than immigrants supposedly pouring in over the border, and it has also delivered boredom.[10]

The study found that inducing boredom by giving people a very tedious task leads to a significant polarization of political orientations.[10] The authors contend that it is boredom's tendency to produce a search for meaning which explains the political shifts it induces.

In a further study, Gillian Wilson recently replicated van Tilburg's and Igou's findings that boredom indeed drives people towards more political extremes.[11] But in her study, entitled 'Boredom Is Polarizing: The Effects of Boredom on Ideological Extremes', she also found a particular tendency for boredom to induce extremism amongst conservatives and not liberals.

An intriguing implication for right-of-centre leaders, in the form of Donald Trump and Boris Johnson, might be increased electoral support, which may encourage them to pursue even more authoritarian policies. This viral pandemic may contribute to a political spiral into extremism.

Another recent study, 'Risk-taking increases under boredom',[12] found people prone to boredom reported greater risk-taking across financial, ethical, recreational, and health or safety domains, and a greater likelihood of choosing risky gambles. The research suggested that elevated risk-taking might be due to the erosion of self-control under boredom. The authors conclude that boredom is associated with making riskier decisions.

This suggests that being invited to stay indoors and comply with a host of other anti-contagion measures, if it elevates boredom, may backfire. The bored might be more likely to take risks in terms of breaking rules, and taking chances with their own health. A study[13] published in the academic journal *Social Psychology* provides further evidence for some of these concerns.

One central psychological reason we go on holiday, whether we realise it or not, is that one cure for tedium is a change in environment. But this treatment is denied to us during the pandemic, and we can't even change our scenery by getting out as much as we need to.

Doctors have themselves struggled with cures for boredom, as is evidenced by the publication of a paper entitled 'Psychotherapy with the Boring Patient'.[14] Unlike most of the other references, I won't divulge the name of the particular doctor who wrote this, in case it induces patients to wonder if they specifically inspired the piece. However, in giving away the name of the academic journal where the paper was published, the inescapable implication is that yes, they were based in Canada, so their patients were most likely... Canadian.

The idea that the patient was where the boringness lay is the paramount conundrum; after all, might it be that it was the therapist who was bored? Is the boredom located in our environment, which we like to blame, or is it really something that stems from deep within us?

Here is a brief psychological test that examines your talent for transforming even the most mundane activities into something gripping. Can you think of a way of making running back and forth for hours on end, between two fixed points, separated by 22 yards, riveting?

Some of the answers have already been discussed above, but were you paying attention? There are more clues below before we supply the final answer. Can you get to it yourself before it is supplied to you? (Is this in itself an anti-boredom tactic?)

Strategies focusing on improving the psychological rewards of work to combat boredom are globally termed 'job enrichment'. At the heart of this approach is the understanding that the most motivated people in the world tend to strive extremely hard for non-financial reasons: they are often relentless, even in the face of poor rewards (that is how we recognise them as being motivated). Deeply motivated people are also those who work hard even if no one is checking up on them.

Job enrichment[8] requires you to start considering your strengths – what particular aspects of your job are you especially good at? It is likely that the more time you can devote to doing these things during your working day, the better you will feel about your job.

A useful exercise is therefore to focus on reorganising your job so that you play to your personal strengths.[7] If this helps you enjoy going to work, in the long run this is better for your colleagues and the people you serve.

Job enrichment also involves workers understanding themselves better, and their managers acknowledging and accepting individual worker's strengths and weaknesses and using this to help people form a deeper connection with their work.

An excellent example of 'job enrichment' principles being used in an innovative way to cure boredom comes from Buckingham Town Cricket Club,[15] who were confronted with the problem of not being allowed to play cricket due to pandemic government restrictions.

Cricket was the last sport to be allowed to recommence after lockdown, and it was soon stopped again due to more government restrictions, leading to a brutally short season.

But Buckingham Town cricket players came up with the idea of a record attempt in aid of charity, after seeing a Guinness World Record completed involving swimming lengths of a pool.[15] There was no ball, it was simply a case of running between the wickets, as happens in the real game of cricket, but in the charity run between wickets, players wore pads and carried a bat.

The community didn't stop sprinting until they shattered the world record for the number of runs completed in twelve hours; indeed they achieved more than double the 3,000 or so it needed to break the record.[15] Almost 200 local people, including the local MP and the town's mayor, took part in the attempt.

The official entry in the book of Guinness World Records[15] now states:

> The most cricket runs in 12 hours (team) is 6,805, achieved by Buckingham Town Cricket Club (UK), in Buckingham, UK, on 30 August 2020 ... The event was organised to raise funds for charity and achieve something amazing. The team covered a total distance of 149,710 yards (136,894 metres).

They intuitively used the principles of combatting boredom. They set a time limit within which a lot had to happen, which in itself made the relatively mundane activity of running back and forth more inherently interesting. They also set a competitive target, which put them under pressure, linked it to a social or community goal that would benefit others, and played to their strengths, namely running between wickets. They were not allowed to do that in a game, so they did it another way. They transformed the inherently boring activity into a high-stakes challenge with an outcome that now mattered not just to any one individual but to the entire group.

This is a functional, socially responsible way of handling boredom. But there is another approach, and it may be closer to explaining what happened to the Pope's Instagram account.

A novel published in 1971, *The Dice Man*, which sold over two million copies and was translated in twenty-three languages, was so controversial in its solution to boredom that it was banned in several countries.[16] Mystery shrouded whether this was a memoir, autobiography or just a made-up story as the author, Luke Rhinehart, a North American psychiatrist, was also the protagonist.

Bored with life, he believes the solution is to introduce radical unpredictability by ceasing to make his own decisions about what to do next, and instead to rely on the roll of a dice. Before he rolls it he assigns a different option to each number and resolves that, whatever shows up, he must perform that action. Life now becomes a game of chance.[16]

One flaw with the concept of the book rapidly becomes apparent, in that being the psychopathic character he is (see Chapter 10 on psychopaths and sex) he tends to assign a suspiciously large number of the options to sexual adventures.

In other words, he was loading the dice before it was rolled. Sure enough, more and more extremes are added to the dice as options, including rape and even murder.

The best-selling book began to gather followers, including the business tycoon Richard Branson, who claimed to be following the way of the dice. Communities subscribing to this philosophy of life were reputed to be forming all over the planet. Rolling the dice became a fixture, apparently, at wife-swapping parties.[16]

In *Diceworld*, a 1999 Channel 4 TV documentary, journalist Ben Marshall took up the challenge of following Luke Rhinehart's philosophy, winding up trying heroin and picking up gay men in Santa Monica. The journalist apparently abandoned the filmed experiment in the end, as he felt following the dice was driving him slowly insane.[16]

The documentary featured a shadowy figure referred to as Luke Rhinehart who admonished the viewers,

> You lead a dull life, a life of slavery, a life that doesn't satisfy you, but there's a way to get out of it. This way is the dice. Let yourself go, submit yourself to it, and you'll see, your life will change, you'll become someone you can't even imagine.

However, it turns out Luke Rhinehart never existed, and instead was the product of the imagination of George Cockcroft, a mild-mannered English teacher who lived a surprisingly unadventurous yet satisfying life in upstate New York, where he raised children and stayed faithfully married for sixty-four years.[16]

There is, however, one postscript to the story which is often neglected. Cockcroft only asked out his future wife, Ann, an attractive nurse he spotted while working as a young man at the same hospital, because he had begun using the roll of a dice to decide what to do on a Saturday night. On one fateful occasion the dice told him to approach her for a game of tennis. He did what the dice instructed, and ended up staying married to her for the rest of his life.[16]

The dice man did roll the dice, but he also knew when to stop gambling.

I believe the essential psychological take-away is usually missed from the story of *The Dice Man*, and there is one in there that can benefit us all. It is in generating the six different options before you roll the dice that the key creative work is done. This creates possibilities which deliver the chance of breaking with boredom. Also, as you consider your options, this assists in self-reflection over your available choices in life.

In fact, I do advocate rolling the dice as a solution to the burden of lockdown boredom. But I also insist you know when *not* to tempt fortune.

There is another solution, which could be viewed as almost the polar opposite of that in *The Dice Man*. This is illustrated in the Hollywood movie that tackles the issue of the inherent boringness of everyday life, *Groundhog Day*, starring Bill Murray and written by Harold Ramis and Danny Rubin. Even today, the most common way to describe wearily how each day under lockdown has been experienced is that it felt like 'Groundhog Day'.

The plot concerns a TV weatherman presenter, Phil Connors, making a short film about the groundhog weather festival in a remote town.

He reluctantly embarks on the day trip, emboldened by the prospect of seducing Rita, his producer, played by the gorgeous Andie MacDowell.[17] However, after shooting the dull, short clip, he finds his plans to return to the big city thwarted as he is mysteriously trapped in the most boring, parochial small town in 'hick-land' USA. For some peculiar reason, he is condemned to repeat the same ostensibly boring day, again and again, without any variation whatsoever.

He transitions through a variety of emotional reactions: first bewilderment, then (being a man) figuring how to manipulate the situation to his own ends, but even this gets boring after a while, so he gradually spirals into despair, and eventually suicidal anguish. He then embarks on a series of suicide attempts.

However, it is at this point that his frustration increases further, because he mysteriously finds himself alive and well at the beginning of the same day yet again. So ultimate liberation from the tedium of life, though seeking fatal oblivion, is itself closed to him. This forces him to try one final fling of the dice: he will confide the bizarre predicament to his producer, Rita, and pray she has some solution. He doesn't have much hope. 'You're a producer, think of something,'[7] he pleads.

In order to prove to Rita that he really has been repeating the same day again and again, Bill Murray's character then relates the life stories of some diners, in front of them, to a startled and embarrassed Rita. He describes details that it would be impossible for him to have gleaned in just the one day's visit that Rita believes is the only time that has elapsed during their twenty-four hours together in the town.

Convinced that something is indeed up, she begs the Bill Murray character to stop, exclaiming that this must be some kind of trick. Bill Murray's character's response is a throwaway line, but it disguises a huge amount of wisdom.

'Well maybe the real God uses tricks, you know? Maybe he's not omnipotent. He's just been around so long he knows everything.'[17]

Rita says later, 'Sometimes I wish I had a thousand lifetimes. I don't know, Phil. Maybe it's not a curse. Just depends on how you look at it.'[17]

Yes, it all does depend on how you look at it.

Because the film's plot does not allow Bill Murray's character to escape from the monotony of the same day again and again, he learns, eventually, painfully, but for the first time, how to make it work. How to derive meaning and satisfaction from that which constrains him. Before, he could always distract himself from the inevitable repetitive nature of life. Once there is no escape, he is forced to confront something he has never faced before, and in so doing he finally breaks through and re-discovers how to live life fully.

The pandemic and the lockdown forced us to come up against ourselves in a way we had never had to before. To survive meant to seize the opportunity, as opposed to complaining that there were not the usual distractions to keep us from facing up to ourselves.

Professor Bhalendu S. Vaishnav commented on the solution to world-weariness in response to one of my articles[18] published in the *British Medical Journal* on boredom in doctors:

A famous saint and philosopher from India, Sri Aurobindo, has said, 'It is only by a constant inner growth that a constant newness can be found in life. There is no other satisfying way.'

8

THE PEOPLE WHO HAVE SPENT TWENTY YEARS PREPARING FOR CORONAVIRUS

Is there one insanity that will help you survive the pandemic, or is any obsession dangerous?

Howard Hughes was an eccentric billionaire who suffered from such an extreme form of obsessive-compulsive disorder that he was reputed to wear tissue boxes on his feet to avoid touching anyone and anything. He may well have suffered from possibly the severest germ phobia on record. So, if he was alive today, would he say I *told* you so?

Think of the very worst lockdown restrictions you could possibly imagine. Now understand that some people, Howard Hughes in particular, actively choose to devote their whole lives to living exactly like that – even when there is ostensibly no pandemic at large in the world beyond.

There is therefore at least one possible irrationality, one possible insanity, that might actually be useful in order to help us survive the pandemic.

Is it now more rational to be wracked with contamination fears?

Is it possible that even if you didn't think you became more OCD during the pandemic, you did, but unconsciously so? If you want to go looking for the unconscious, dreams are a good place to search.

Dr Natalia Bezerra Mota[1] deployed computerised technology to analyse the words people used when describing their dreams.

Dream content from before the COVID-19 outbreak was compared to that during Brazil's lockdown in March and April 2020. The analysis found that words suggesting sadness and anger were now more frequent, and also words related to 'contamination' and 'cleanliness' occurred much more often.

Sigmund Freud, the pioneer of the notion that our emotional problems largely arise from unconscious conflicts, placed great store in analysing dreams. He believed the unconscious squirreled away secrets into our nightly visions, which it was trying to hide from our conscious awareness. According to Freud and his followers, you could only achieve true release from mental agony by grasping what was lurking in your unconscious. Interpreting these visions which come to us in our sleep, however, has now fallen out of favour in modern psychology clinics; it's no longer viewed as particularly scientific, more akin to reading tea leaves left at the bottom of a cup. But the findings of this latest study were based on a possibly more systematic scrutiny because, in a sense, it was the computer which was really analysing the dream.

The study suggests that even if you appear outwardly calm in the face of the contagion, anxieties could be surfacing in your dreams, particularly fears over contamination and cleanliness. Maybe you have become more concerned about these issues than you realised.

Given there is a particular psychiatric disorder which focuses on fears over contamination, and harbours constant cleanliness doubts, this raises the real question of whether the pandemic has pushed more people into this particular disorder, consciously or unconsciously, compared with any other. But how to find out, if that means we need to go searching through your unconscious?

How would you respond if questioned by a psychologist as to whether 'handling wet and slimy things' upset you?

If you were asked that question, you may have inadvertently slipped into a time machine and found yourself transported back to the heyday of Freudian psychoanalytic thinking, which dominated psychology and psychiatry in the 1950s and 1960s.

That particular inquiry was part of a psychoanalytic test attempting to measure just how 'anal' you were.

At the beginning of the twentieth century, Sigmund Freud claimed to have discovered a profoundly powerful cluster of personality traits, which became infamous as the 'anal triad'. The so-called anal-retentive personality was rigid, overly orderly, pedantic, obsessed with cleanliness, obstinate, stubborn, and mean with money. The triad was orderliness, obstinacy and parsimony.

Freud contended these personality features clustered in those who may have become fixated on defecation during childhood toilet training. They may have got some kind of perverse pleasure in either emptying their bowels or in 'holding back'.

As you might imagine, attempting to conduct scientific psychology experiments which explored this theory had its challenges. Here is an example of one such study, entitled 'An action test of hypotheses concerning the anal personality', published in the *Journal of Abnormal Psychology* in 1966.[2] The experiment involved the psychologists asking the subjects taking part in the experiment to submerge their arm up to the elbow in a bucket filled with a substance designed to replicate the feel and smell of excrement. While they reached into the pail they had to use their hands to identify objects at the bottom!

Here is an excerpt from the methodology of the experiment as published in the journal:

> The subject's task required that he immerse his arm, up to the elbow, into a bucket filled with water at room temperature which was hidden from his view by a curtain. Three irregularly shaped flat bits of aluminium, larger than those commonly used in jigsaw puzzles, had been dropped by the experimenter to the bottom of the bucket. A card with the outlines of six such pieces was displayed in full view of the subject. The instruction was to explore the contours of the three pieces, one after another, and to decide as quickly as possible to which of the displayed outlines it corresponded. The subject was required to leave his arm immersed until he had reached a decision. Then he was to remove the piece and place it on the table beside the bucket so that the experimenter might record the results. Four trials of three judgments each were administered using water as a medium. This was followed by four trials in a mixture of used crankcase oil and two pounds of flour. This dirty and odorous medium was assumed to arouse anxieties and other responses similar to those commonly attached to faeces.[2]

The results of the experiment confirmed that those measured to be more 'anal-retentive' personalities struggled to perform the task as well as low anal scorers.

Why on earth are we discussing this here?

Because, having been discarded by mainstream psychology for decades, the anal personality type saw a revival in interest directly because of COVID-19. After finding itself languishing for decades 'in the toilet', so to speak, the virus seemed to flush it back to the surface again.

At the beginning of the pandemic, in the Western world, the demand for toilet paper went through the roof, with some retailers reporting an increase of up to 700 per cent in sales. Despite official appeals to refrain from panic purchasing, supermarkets across the world faced toilet paper shortages. The resulting scarcity led to pipes clogging after some were forced to use alternatives to toilet paper.

A study[3] investigated the psychological drivers to toilet paper hoarding by surveying 1,029 adults from thirty-five countries.

The authors argue that the personality characteristic most people would associate with stockpiling would be selfishness. Another theory was that those who are more sensitive to disgust in times of a spreading disease might find accumulating toilet paper as somehow comforting. It might serve as a symbol of safety, therefore alleviating the perceived threat.

Consequently, stockpiling toilet paper during the COVID-19 pandemic would be predicted to be found particularly among those who feel especially threatened by the virus.

Finally, stockpiling toilet paper has also been interpreted in terms of classic Freudian psychoanalytic theory. The notorious Freudian idea that there is an 'anal-retentive personality', characterised by orderliness and self-discipline, might be particularly inclined to hoard toilet paper.

The study found that Europeans shopped for toilet paper more frequently than North American residents, but still ended up with less toilet paper in stock. Europeans seemed to be running on some kind of toilet paper treadmill. The authors resolved the paradox by pointing out that on average, toilet paper rolls come in bigger packages in the USA (up to thirty-six rolls per package) than in most European countries (eight to sixteen rolls). Perhaps the average US citizen's weekly shop looks to a European like stockpiling for a nuclear winter.

The study[3] found that the perceived threat of COVID-19 as well as emotionality, or the tendency to worry a lot and feel anxious, plus conscientiousness, or being more long-sighted, self-controlled and more orderly, all predict heightened toilet paper stockpiling behaviour.

The authors conclude that toilet paper functions as a subjective symbol of safety.

If you are visiting someone you don't know very well, perhaps you are considering dating them, and you open one of their cupboards inadvertently, and piles of rolls of toilet paper fall out, then you now know you can predict something about their personality. They will tend to be somewhat 'anal', orderly and conscientious.

Peter Goffin, a long-term sufferer from obsessive-compulsive disorder (OCD) who appears to have routinely individually disinfected each item of his grocery shopping as soon as he got home, confided to the BBC that he may have spent twenty years preparing for the current pandemic.[4] Goffin explained that millions of people around the world are only now asking themselves questions such as: 'Did that person in the shop get too close to me? Did I wash my hands for long enough? Will this soap kill all the germs?' Yet sufferers from OCD, such as himself, agonised in exactly this way over germs as part of everyday life long before the pandemic arrived. They developed rituals, like counting during repetitive hand-washing, designed to keep at bay the fear that they had become contaminated.

Goffin told the BBC that in his experience, anecdotally, many people with pre-existing anxiety over germs are now less anxious during the current pandemic, maybe because they don't feel so alone with their obsessions anymore.

That syndrome, which now seems to have added benefits, is to be so obsessional that you might have attracted the pejorative label of 'control freak' before. While sufferers can endure a wide variety of symptoms, fixations over contamination and incessant handwashing are in fact some of the most common.

Dr Debanjan Banerjee has published an investigation entitled 'The other side of COVID-19: Impact on obsessive compulsive disorder (OCD) and hoarding', suggesting that the pandemic may have a specific impact on OCD above all other emotional conditions.[5]

In his argument he points out that the demand for sanitizers, soaps and gloves has sky-rocketed, as compulsive handwashing is now considered to be an essential precaution against catching the virus. Public health officials emphasise the importance of sterilising measures, including repetitive cleaning, as well as vigilance against contamination.[5]

OCD victims always harbour doubts over whether ordinary hygiene is really good enough and have always felt compelled to decontaminate.

One possible mental impact of the pandemic might be to make 'normal' people a bit more OCD, while obsessionals might adapt better to the post-COVID world than the sloppier amongst us. We may be entering the era of OCD.

Are they are going to feel vindicated and superior?

Profound changes to our lives include not just more handwashing but even a minimum duration recommended for it, which is very OCD. Ritualistic patterns we are encouraged to embrace include repetitive handwashing steps: precisely the kind of rituals obsessionals swear by. Intrusively prompting others to observe strict hygiene measures, while becoming suspicious that surfaces surrounding you have been contaminated by an unseen germ, all appear to come straight out of the OCD playbook. Then there is the hoarding of masks, soaps, sanitizers, disinfectants and toilet paper.

But just before you leave (don't touch the door handles on the way out please) with the impression that the pandemic has produced OCD nirvana, in fact it is also possible that the obsessional could be more de-stabilised by all of the above.

How to stay balanced in a world of increasing OCD remains the essential question.

Referred to by French doctors as '*la folie du doute*', or the madness of doubt, OCD lies at the heart of everyone's new anxiety over an invisible threat which might be infecting us, unawares, right now. Harbouring doubt over whether you got infected or not, or took an unnecessary risk, is inevitable.

The correct coping skill is to learn how to handle these misgivings and to distinguish productive doubt from unhealthy rumination. If you obsessively protect yourself from contamination, it is also possible to slip over to the dark side and become too obsessional, on a slide which can lead ultimately to some of the most extreme forms of madness recorded.

How *would* Howard Hughes cope? And is his story a caution to us at this precise moment? If by the end of his life Hughes was so afraid of germs that he withdrew from the world, did that mean it was a stable strategy – in other words, an approach to life that actually worked?[6]

Think of Howard Hughes and, for most people, the enduring image of a shabby, reclusive eccentric comes to mind. Open any biography of the legendary film-maker and you will read about any number of Hughes's extraordinary behavioural tics; so much so that his name is now synonymous with the stereotypical oddball billionaire.

By 1966, at the age of sixty, Hughes was reputedly the world's wealthiest man, but by then he had such a terror of contagious disease that he avoided contact with anyone if at all possible. Only his security guards and doctors saw him. He was injecting codeine, and had moved to Mexico to get hold of it more readily. He broke needles in his arms, which later showed up on autopsy X-rays. He shunned clothing and let his hair and nails grow. His teeth rotted and fell out because he never brushed them. He never bathed. He urinated on the floor, but might sit on the toilet for twenty hours at a time because of extreme constipation as a result of the codeine addiction.

This paradox of living in excrement and dirt while suffering from germophobia is well known to psychiatrists; it is even referred to in some research papers as the 'Howard Hughes dilemma'. It is explained by the irrational fear of dirt becoming so intense that no amount of cleaning is seen to be good enough, and therefore cleaning is eventually abandoned altogether.

Hughes deteriorated physically and lost so much weight that his staff thought he would die. Spending hours cleaning every nearby surface, he discarded his clothes and remained nude (except for shoes, and sometimes a shirt) for the rest of his life. In 1976, on his way to a Houston hospital, he died, apparently of heart failure. His estate at the time was valued at $650 million.

Howard Hughes was born in 1905. He was an only child and the object of excessive concern from his mother, who herself almost died at birth. He was born at a time when polio was rife and awareness of the disease would have been high. His mother's fear of germs underscored his childhood. She was obsessively protective, and his father was frequently absent, which may have driven her to an overly intense and protective relationship with her only child. After Howard suffered a mysterious paralysis in later adolescence, his parents were desperately afraid that he might indeed have the dreaded polio, and brought a physician from New York to care for him full-time. Hughes would grow used to commanding personal attention from doctors.

The most painful events of his life occurred when his mother died during minor surgery when he was sixteen and, two years later, when his father died of a heart attack during a business meeting. This second sudden death would have traumatised Hughes, and resulted in a period of depression, over-concern with his health and increased social withdrawal.

Clearly, the loss of the only two people with whom he had close relationships deepened his fears of death and increased his vulnerability to later psychological dysfunction. It would have been only natural that Hughes should become preoccupied with the possibility of any innocuous symptom being a harbinger of death. His growing fear of germs as a young man suggests the start of an obsessive-compulsive disorder.

Obsessions are persistent, recurrent and distressing thoughts – such as the possibility of dying. Compulsions are repetitive behaviours designed to protect against a future situation – such as catching an infectious illness.

At eighteen, Hughes took over the family business in Houston. He would finally have found something over which he could feel mastery, and he would have set out compulsively to obtain more. It was clear to those who knew him that his ambitions were high – to be the richest man alive, and a top film producer and aviator. He managed all three, winning world fame in his early twenties. Yet he seemed embarrassed and uneasy with the visibility that this entailed. He dated famous actresses, but seemed more interested in collecting them than establishing serious relationships. Many elements of OCD manifest here; such people focus on worst-case scenarios and work to eliminate even the minutest chance of mistakes, while Hughes's 'collecting' of women indicates the strong need for control over his environment.

I think the profound problem a clinician would encounter treating someone as successful as Hughes would have been persuading him that there was actually anything fundamentally wrong with him. After all, by his early twenties he had produced *Two Arabian Knights*, which won an Academy Award, and he would go on to create a number of classics. As a pilot, he set cross-country and round-the-world speed records. And the income from the business he inherited provided him with almost unlimited funds.

Another problem would be that he could, at the click of a finger, summon a new therapist with a different evaluation. If I were treating him I would insist that I would be his only physician and only source of prescriptions. To ensure an uninterrupted supply of codeine, he played his doctors against each other. But would my therapeutic manoeuvre be interpreted with suspicion by those who were afraid of losing their influence over Hughes?

The issue of control is at the heart of OCD. Hughes was able to evade psychological expertise and treatment so completely because he could use his power and wealth to get others to carry out his elaborate rituals – waving newspapers to scare away imaginary flies, opening doors with their feet to avoid touching the knobs, putting tape around windows, and washing their hands and everything else in sight.

The tragedy at the heart of Hughes's life is that he paid doctors simply to supply him with codeine to feed his addiction, but they never insisted he face up to his OCD. Would a modern psychiatrist fare any better against the manipulative billionaire?

A study[7] published in the prestigious *American Journal of Psychiatry* appears to be the most comprehensive and detailed examination of obsessive-compulsive disorder in a Western community. The study is part of a longitudinal investigation of the health and behaviour of all the children born during a one-year period in 1972–73 in Dunedin, New Zealand.

The first astonishing finding from this unique study is that while the prevalence of a formal OCD diagnosis is just 2.4 per cent at age twenty-six and 1.8 per cent at age thirty-two, the investigators found that 21–25 per cent of the cohort (including 13–17 per cent of those without a mental disorder) reported obsessions and/or compulsions at those ages. These very high rates are also consistent with findings from another major study of a community elsewhere in the Western world, so it looks like these high rates really do reflect the fact that serious OCD symptoms are extremely common in the general public.

31–42 per cent of the general public with no diagnosed mental disorder reported having been bothered by obsessions for periods of over two weeks, 25 per cent reported experiencing obsessions for more than an hour a day, and approximately 15 per cent reported being emotionally upset by them.

Regarding compulsions, 33–45 per cent of the whole cohort reported performing them for periods of over two weeks; 11–12 per cent of healthy individuals reported being upset by having to perform such rituals.

In his accompanying editorial in the *American Journal of Psychiatry* commenting on this important study, Dr Murray Stein[6] suggests we should be asking, 'What, in addition to the propensity to have obsessive-compulsive symptoms (which are common), leads to expression of OCD (which is rare)?'

Suffering from an OCD symptom was strongly predictive of developing other psychological problems. OCD symptomatology is clearly very corrosive to your mental health. For example, another critical finding from this study[7] is that suffering from a cluster of obsessive-compulsive symptoms was strongly associated with other anxiety and mood disorders.

That these supposedly counter-productive aspects of behaviour can endure for so long, and even begin in childhood, raises naturally the question of whether they are somehow under genetic control; indeed it also follows from that theory that they may have an evolutionary benefit.

Is it possible that hundreds of thousands of years ago, in dirtier and more dangerous, chaotic times, those of us who washed and checked and ordered things more than usual were at an evolutionary advantage compared to less fastidious, more careless individuals? Hoarding is a classic OCD symptom; is it beyond the bounds of possibility that hoarding at times when famine was not infrequent and life more precarious was of benefit to survival?

As a General Adult Psychiatry clinician working at the interface between primary care and referrals to secondary care, I am personally familiar with high levels of OCD remaining untreated in the community, or held solely within primary care. This experience leads me to tentatively advocate a model which accounts for when those suffering from OCD for many years finally 'transition' into seeking formal psychiatric care.

For me there is a common underlying theme here: the issue of *control*. And this is something we may need to take on board as part of the mental vaccine for COVID-19.

I contend that those with OCD experiences will finally be prompted to seek help when they believe that they are now verging on an inability to control their symptoms.

The paradox at the heart of OCD, I believe, is that control over various aspects of their lives and their minds is much more important for this group than for the general population. This value in itself produces distress; yet on top of this they also frequently adopt strategies which are only precariously successful.

The pandemic is a uniquely stressful event because it directly attacks – on several fronts – our sense of control over our lives.

Before the current government and media campaign to get us to be more careful about washing our hands, in fact, psychiatrists were very familiar with a group of people who were already very concerned about whether they had cleaned or purified enough. Indeed, this section of society probably washed their hands excessively. These people suffered from so-called 'contamination' fears which are a well-known symptom of OCD, as we described in the previous section.

Contamination anxiety is an intense persistent feeling of having been polluted, infected and endangered because of contact, no matter how mild or innocuous, with a person or location or object that is viewed as soiled, impure, infectious or harmful. Feeling contaminated is accompanied by fear, disgust, feeling dirty and shame.

Is there likely to be a particular impact on Asians in the UK? Asians may be more likely to be self-employed and might live more closely together as extended families, so all these factors could have particular implications for them in the current economic climate.

But perhaps the most surprising psychological difference between Asians and the rest of the UK population may come from an unexpected source – the sink.

A new study entitled 'Examination of racial differences in assessment of OCD symptoms and obsessive beliefs'[7] has confirmed that there are significant racial differences between Caucasians, Asians, Hispanics and Blacks in terms of their general fears of contamination.

The research found that Asians scored higher than other racial groups for fears of contamination, arguably in an attempt to compensate for possible racial prejudice over cleanliness, perhaps historically, as regarding Asian food and other aspects of Asian culture.

Within the Asian population, among those who are already prone to being more obsessional, with a dread of contamination and living with washing/cleaning compulsions, these fears have been shown to manifest themselves significantly more frequently in Indian women than in men.

A study entitled 'Gender differences in obsessive-compulsive disorder: Findings from a large Indian sample'[8] also found that these more obsessional Indian women suffered elevated suicide risk compared to obsessional Indian men, suggesting that excessive contamination fears contribute to poorer mental health.

But a major flaw with the media approach on how to cope with the stress of the pandemic is to suggest that doing away with anxiety is the correct approach.

In fact, a certain amount of apprehension is healthy, particularly if it leads you to take precautions and avoid dangerous predicaments. Those who suffer from what might be considered excessive contamination fears may just now be, paradoxically, the ones finding it easiest to survive the quarantine.

Anxiety, when it is justified, can keep you alive.

On the other hand, excessive anxiety can be just as dangerous.[9] Those with excessive contamination fears can even irrationally avoid a life-saving vaccination because they fear contamination from something being injected into their body. They court the risk of falling victim to a dangerous infection without the protection of the vaccination, despite all that excessive handwashing.

Asians are more likely to die from COVID-19 compared with other ethnic groups, yet according to the Royal Society for Public Health only 57 per cent of those with black, Asian and minority ethnic (BAME) backgrounds are presently likely to accept a vaccine, compared to 79 per cent of white respondents; confidence was lowest in Asians, with 55 per cent likely to agree to take the jab.[10]

Ethnic minorities also distrusted previous vaccines: the Human Papilloma Virus vaccine and the flu jab had much lower take-up among ethnic minorities. Influenza vaccination rates across the whole of Asia are low compared to the West.

The press speculation as to why there is such widespread 'vaccine hesitancy' among Asians seems to centre on a supposed tendency for those from ethnic minority backgrounds to favour more alternative or herbal remedies, from their traditional backgrounds, and so reject Western medicine. But the vaccine scepticism of Asians may also be a symptom of a deeper, more fundamental mindset difference about trust in general. Ethnic minorities have been shown again and again in various scientific studies of Western societies to have much less confidence in others, including institutions and other people, significantly less than the majority ethnic group, in this case white people.

Asians don't just trust vaccines less; they have less trust in practically everything.

Professor of Criminal Justice Sandra Susan Smith recently showed in her research[11] that the three most powerful determinants of trust are education level (the more educated tend to trust more); age (older people tend to trust more); and race. Of all of these, race is the most powerful of all in determining how much you trust others, as explained in her study entitled 'Race and Trust'. Ethnic minorities trust less.

Just how powerful race is in explaining trust levels is shown in the finding that in the USA, trust among the wealthiest blacks was similar to levels of trust expressed by the poorest whites.

Ethnic minorities are believed to trust so little in comparison with whites because of the bruising and repeated experience of discrimination. This makes it difficult for them to have faith in others, though they do tend to trust members of their community more.

This tendency to be somewhat distrustful may have been transformed into a secret strength in the community. Asian children outperformed other ethnic groups educationally because their parents pushed them with the threat that to get a job in a prejudiced society they'd have to be significantly better than the competition.

Asians chose to be entrepreneurs and run their own businesses rather than work for others, as they placed little confidence in working their way up through workplace politics. There wasn't going to be fair treatment and promotion from managers not of their ethnicity.

But now this lack of trust could come back to haunt the Asian community if widespread distrust of the vaccine leads to poor take-up and therefore continued higher mortality rates.

The inherent problem of being suspicious of the outside world and as a result remaining insular and self-contained is that you are deprived of learning opportunities to figure out who and when to trust. If you only ever work for yourself or go for job interviews with far and away the best qualifications, you never find out if you could have trusted the outside world, so mistrust becomes a self-fulfilling prophecy which never gets dispelled.

Let's take an example: if you never lend anyone money, because you just assume no one is ever going to pay you back, as you don't trust anyone, then you will never learn whom you can lend to, and whom you can't.

Many Asians, despite having made the UK their home, remain surprisingly cut off from it, because of this deep tendency to be suspicious of outsiders.

If mistrust means you never take the first step into the unknown then how to break this cycle?

The company which pioneered the Pfizer vaccine, BioNTech, has as its CEO Dr Uğur Şahin, who was born in Turkey and immigrated to Germany, where he is a professor of experimental oncology, and now one of Germany's 100 wealthiest people, worth over

$5 billion dollars. His wife, Özlem Türeci, co-founder and chief medical officer of BioNTech, was born in Germany but has Turkish parents. This tendency to marry others from the same ethnic background in first-generation immigrants may have something to do with mistrust of the host community. As an Asian, if you don't trust much, you may at least believe in the excellence and hard work that could lie behind these two exemplars of immigrant success.

You just took part in a little informal psychology experiment: now you know the origin of this vaccine has something to do with immigrants, has that changed how much you trust the jab?

Yet it remains the case that fears of contamination in the widest sense run deep, and are possibly even genetically wired into our brains.[12]

We all need just the right level of anxiety in order to survive. Too much can be as harmful as too little. Moreover, as we have seen in this chapter, we also need to be aware when it is possible our culture, or even our race, pushes us too far in one direction or another.

It turns out racial bias, and a host of other prejudices against those different from us, may arise from the same deep psychological origins as contamination fears. A pandemic, in triggering widespread distaste for uncleanness, could widen fissures between different groups who already harbour a distaste for each other. Was it really a coincidence that the Second World War, a conflict that had something to do with anxiety over racial purity, came just twenty years after the Spanish Flu?

9

IS THE PANDEMIC LEADING TO A NEW NORMAL OF REVENGE PORN?

No kissing may lead to bad choices

A study conducted by Canadian researcher Samantha Bates[1] into the experiences of victims of revenge porn reported the following case. A victim's (now ex-)husband brought her to a hotel room and drugged her. She had no memory of what happened, but later found out that he and another man had raped her. She divorced him shortly after, and seven months later, he sent a video containing footage of the rape to the school board where she worked. She was fired from her job as a school superintendent immediately after the video was sent to her colleagues, and the police were still investigating the rape at the time of the interview.

Under the headline 'Revenge porn new normal', after cases surged in lockdown, the BBC News website reported on the recent dramatic rise in reports of so-called revenge porn. The problem has apparently been exacerbated by enforced social isolation.

Revenge porn occurs when a resentful, often rejected, person uploads revealing pictures of someone online, often as retaliation following the end of a relationship.

The BBC explains that there has been a 22 per cent rise in reports from victims made to a UK government-funded helpline compared with last year. The charity has helped remove 22,515 revenge porn images this year. The BBC even claims there are now fears that the rising epidemic of revenge porn is becoming 'the new normal'.[2]

The report also revealed that recent research by UK domestic violence charity Refuge found that one in seven young women has received threats that intimate photos will be disseminated without their consent.

Perhaps the issue of rising levels of revenge porn illuminates a largely hidden problem with the pandemic, which is that it may have disrupted intimate connections in all sorts of unexpected ways.

In an academic study entitled 'Revenge Porn and Mental Health: A Qualitative Analysis of the Mental Health Effects of Revenge Porn on Female Survivors', Samantha Bates[1] conducted in-depth interviews with eighteen female revenge porn survivors. One of the victims interviewed in this study

> ... changed her routines and behaviours when she was alone due to strangers showing up at her house looking for sex after seeing naked photos of her on the Internet. Her ex-boyfriend used internet chat rooms and pretended to be her online. He would send naked photos of her to strangers, give them her home address, and ask them to come over to her house for sex. She mentioned one time in particular when a man broke into her house, grabbed her, and tried to choke her.

Another study entitled 'The dark side of the online self: A pragmatist critique of the growing plague of revenge porn'[3] reports that several non-consensual pornography websites encourage users to submit compromising images of ex-partners for revenge. These websites often encourage others to then leave insulting comments. For example, in one three-month period, one revenge porn website received 10,000 photo submissions.

A further study,[4] entitled 'Criminalizing revenge porn' and published in the *Wake Forest Law Review*, examined 1,244 non-consensual pornography survivors and found that more than 50 per cent of survivors' full names and links to social media profiles accompanied the naked photos, and that 20 per cent of survivors' email addresses and phone numbers were posted with their photos.

Impacts of non-consensual pornography include public disgrace, the loss of new romantic partners, depression and anxiety, job loss, difficulties securing new employment, and offline harassment and stalking.[1]

Previous research has established that women generally do not send nude photos to men they do not know. Samantha Bates argues in her study that a level of trust is likely necessary before women feel comfortable sending a nude photo. This outlook counters, she contends, the 'she should have known better' argument.[1]

Some more of the participants' experiences with revenge porn, from the study by Samantha Bates,[1] are included below.

Her ex-boyfriend posted an eBay auction for a disc containing naked photos of her, which she successfully had taken down from eBay. However, a year later, he created a porn website with the naked photos of her, which included her full name, the name of her town, the name of the college she taught at, and a solicitation saying, *hot for teacher? Come get it.*

Another victim's ex-boyfriend

… set up hidden cameras around her home, and she ended the relationship shortly after discovering he was secretly filming her. After she broke up with him, he created a website and several social media pages using unflattering and nude photos of her from the footage.

Another victim spoke through tears as she told her story of the impact revenge porn had on her mental health:

When the actual video was released, um, well, I can admit now that I was suicidal, and … to let you know how suicidal I was, I didn't tell anybody because I knew if I told anyone that I just wanted to kill myself that they would try to stop me, so I didn't tell anyone because I didn't want anyone to stop me … I lost my reputation … financially I'm ruined, I lost my career, a 25-year stellar career … I had a doctorate degree. I lost everything. So, how did that make me feel? Um, devastated. I just don't even have words to describe it. Horrifying, humiliated, embarrassed, betrayed, I mean, I just never thought that a man I had loved, I married him, he was my husband, I trusted him. How could he do something like this?

This study uncovered profound impacts on victims including suicidality, PTSD, anxiety and depression. The research revealed striking similarities between the mental health effects of sexual assault and revenge porn for survivors, suggesting that revenge porn should be classified as a sexual offence.

Standard advice on how to prevent revenge porn includes that women should not send naked photos if they have been in a relationship with the recipient for less than a year, and to only send explicit shots if their face is not in the image.[1]

It would appear there need to be more legal resources, including laws in place to help those who have been affected by revenge porn. The police should be required take it more seriously, and not judge or shame victims.

Yet the horrendous stories of lives ruined uncovered by this recent research suggests maybe even deeper changes are required in our society, including, perhaps, addressing the shame culture surrounding women's bodies as well as the various forms of male violence and coercion women face.[1]

Another issue raised by the rise of revenge porn during the pandemic is that if we are prevented from normal ways of conducting relationships, through, for example, physical contact, this might lead to fundamental disturbances in the relationships themselves. Is it possible that our ability to assess who is right for us, for example, is fundamentally disturbed when we can't meet to hug or to kiss?

Rafael Wlodarski and Robin Dunbar recently published one of the most in-depth studies of kissing,[5] involving 308 male and 594 female participants, aged eighteen to sixty-three.

The investigation challenges conventional views of why we kiss. The surprising results suggest there may be more going on beneath the surface, when it comes to kissing, than is commonly realised.

The study concludes that kissing may be so common because it serves a useful biological or evolutionary purpose. It might even have evolved a 'survival of the fittest' function. At a conscious or subconscious level, women in particular are using kissing to assess whether a potential partner is of sufficient quality to mate with.[5]

That there might be more to kissing than meets the eye is suggested by older studies cited by Wlodarski and Dunbar in their paper. For example, previous research has found that men are much more likely to initiate kissing before sex, the theory being that, given the timing, kissing here serves 'arousal' purposes. Yet women are more likely to initiate kissing after sex, where there might be a different intention. At this time 'relationship maintenance' might be the priority.

This 'attachment' theory of kissing, perhaps particularly for women, according to Wlodarski and Dunbar, has previously been suggested by anecdotal evidence from other researchers examining the business practices of working prostitutes. Commercial sex workers often, apparently, refuse to kiss clients on the basis that it is 'too intimate' or 'it smacks too much of genuine desire and love for the other person'.

Scientists speculate that kissing might also signal commitment because of the intimacy of the act. It necessarily requires breaching personal boundaries. Kissers risk various health hazards, including influenza, herpes simplex virus or meningococcal meningitis. These perils indicate there should be a powerful evolutionary or 'survival of the fittest' reason behind kissing, as life might be safer without it. It is also a highly intimate and arousing activity, releasing various neurotransmitters and neuropeptides in the brain thought to be responsible for increased feelings of attachment.

While previous research has found both men and women rate kissing as the form of physical affection 'most expressive of love', women seem to place greater overall importance on romantic kissing than men. In a separate study, about to be published, Wlodarski and Dunbar found that women in the most fertile phase of their menstrual cycle valued kissing most at initial relationship stages.[5]

Men and women may have different reasons to kiss, because evolutionary theory predicts they will deploy various courtship and relationship tactics in different ways. The contrasting mating strategies might be in conflict.

As historically sex was always accompanied by a chance of falling pregnant, requiring much more 'biological' investment from women, it would have a different meaning between sexes. This would imply women should be much more discerning when it comes to selecting a mate, given their higher levels of biological investment.

Wlodarski and Dunbar point to a considerable body of research confirming that females are indeed much more rigorous and selective when it comes to entertaining a possible mate than males. As a result, the experimenters hypothesised that, particularly for women, kissing serves a kind of 'mate-assessment' function.

Their study, 'Examining the Possible Functions of Kissing in Romantic Relationships', found very little evidence the primary purpose of kissing is arousal. Instead, the results indicated kissing serves a useful 'mate-assessment' function. Women placed greater importance on kissing in romantic relationships, and stated that an initial kiss was more likely to affect their attraction to a potential mate than did men. Women were more likely than men to have experienced a change in attraction after an initial kiss.

Both men and women who rated themselves as scoring higher on attractiveness rated kissing as more important than 'low attractiveness' participants. Those who see themselves as more attractive have been previously found to be more selective, and value more cues of genetic quality in mating.

Kissing was also generally seen as more important in long-term relationship contexts (but particularly so by women), and kissing frequency was found to be related to relationship satisfaction.

Women thought kissing was more important than men 'at other times not related to sex'. Overall, for both men and women, kissing was seen as much more important with long-term partners. Both men and women agreed that kissing short-term partners was seen as most important only before sex, less important during sex, even less vital after sex, and least crucial at 'other times'.

Rafael Wlodarski and Robin Dunbar concede that while one of the most obvious consequences of kissing is indeed bodily arousal, their data did not support the widely held belief that getting 'turned on' is the driving factor associated with the prevalence of kissing.

Instead, perhaps the most intriguing and important finding from the study is that kissing could even be as important as sex, if not more important. The investigation found that having a partner who was a 'good' kisser, greater frequency of kissing in the relationship and greater satisfaction with the amount of kissing were all positively associated with relationship quality, while the frequency of sex in the relationship was not significantly related to relationship quality.

The purpose of kissing might depend on where you are in the relationship, during the act. Wlodarski and Dunbar suggest kissing can help both assess mates, and facilitate attachment, at different stages of the relationship.

The authors conclude there may be something unique about romantic kissing that affects attachment and relationship satisfaction to a greater degree than more physiologically arousing activities such as sex.

Men, evolutionary psychologists hypothesise, display an evolved tendency to seek a variety of sexual partners, because ancestral men who did so reproduced more than males who did not. Men therefore evolved to pursue a wider variety of sexual opportunities. Due to being the gender which falls pregnant, breastfeeds and does most infant care, women might have evolved a sexual strategy where they invested more in a smaller number of their own children (whom they can be certain are their own). Evolutionary psychologists predict they are therefore choosier over who their mates.

According to psychologists Martie Haselton and David Buss,[6] the recurrent errors men and women make in determining who truly fancies them are engendered by the consequences of getting things wrong.

The major error for a man would be to miss the fact a woman really did want to sleep with him, so, according to their study, men tend to overestimate sexual intent in women. Haselton and Buss argue that women are also prone to blunder in reading men's romantic intent; they don't spot that a man is truly committed to them. Their study, published in the *Journal of Personality and Social Psychology*, argues that for women the costs of falsely inferring more commitment in a possible partner when little or none exists had more devastating consequences, at least in ancestral conditions, than not seeing commitment when it's there.

Haselton and Buss contend that an ancestral woman who consented to sex with a man who abandoned her shortly thereafter, because of low commitment, suffered the costs of an unwanted or untimely pregnancy, raising children alone, and reputational damage. These costs might hinder survival of the child, and impair future reproductive potential.[6]

An ancestral woman who erred by underestimating a man's commitment, in contrast, might have merely evoked more numerous and frequent displays of dedication by the truly devoted man. Valentine's Day is therefore explained by evolutionary theory.[6]

Given the tremendous evolutionary importance of securing a faithful mate, modern women are descendants of ancestral mothers who erred on the side of caution. Women are therefore 'commitment-sceptics' in the face of men professing their love.

These results could have been contaminated by a fact that psychologists have found for short-term mating: men relax their standards when it comes to physical attractiveness in the opposite sex. In contrast, women, if pursuing a shorter-term fling, *increase* their standards for physical attractiveness in potential mates.

Haselton and Buss caution in their study that even if gender differences are found in seduction, this could still be due to cultural influences such as the media. They point out that men are exposed to media images depicting women as initially coy, but then overcome with sexual desire.[6]

The media and academic research also still seem to largely ignore the lesbian, bisexual, gay and transgender perspective.

But given all the contamination and powerful forces at work from our genes and the media, can we get better at spotting other's real romantic interest?

Haselton and Buss found in their study that men's quantification of their own sisters' sexual interest was lower than their perceptions of other women's erotic objectives. The results suggested that men may perceive their sisters' sexual intent fairly accurately. This was because all the desire and emotion which normally contaminate this assessment had, almost by definition, been removed from the predicament.

Patients confide secrets to their therapists which they won't reveal to anyone else, including best friends, spouses or surveys. My network of clinicians have been reporting a massive upswing in covert promiscuity among their clients during the lockdown. Both genders have been pursuing sex in a more wanton and uninhibited way than ever before, including orgies and multiple partners during one evening. People are acting out of character and appear to be in the grip of strong emotions arising out of the various strains of the pandemic.

These activities have been going on covertly and involve breaking multiple rules over travelling and socialising, so are under the radar of the media and also, perhaps most importantly, those modelling the pandemic.

Not everyone is 'partying', but a significant minority appear to be.

The danger of relationships conducted during the pandemic, beset with obstacles such as lockdowns or social distancing, is that background emotions of frustration or desperation will come to the fore. These will contaminate and maybe even dominate our mental state, adversely influencing our ability to dispassionately assess what is really going on in our intimate lives.

IO

DO PSYCHOPATHS SECURE MORE SEX DESPITE SOCIAL DISTANCING?

The personality type that thrives when ordered to socially isolate

Everyone thinks everyone else is having way more sex than they themselves are. This anxiety may be even more exaggerated during a pandemic.

Peter Florjančič,[1] an inventor and wealthy playboy who died aged 101 in 2020, held at various times over 400 patents, including the perfume spray, the plastic photographic slide frame, and the cigarette lighter used by James Bond in the movies.

He deserted from his conscription into the German Army in 1943, fleeing to Austria. In order to elude the pursuing Gestapo, he disguised himself as a skiing tourist, faking his own death in an avalanche, then slipped into neutral Switzerland. Perhaps this peculiar psychological ingenuity over 'invention' saved his life, and also later made him several fortunes with his gizmos and gadgets.

It was perhaps also within this spirit of invention that he also, apparently, had a habit of playing audio recordings of wild yet never-ending passionate sex very loudly in his hotel room, for hours on end. He would then revel in the reputation he'd established, given the other guests' envious, incredulous glances the next morning.

As I said, everyone thinks everyone else is having way more sex than they themselves are. Especially during a pandemic. I may have some bad news. In some cases it is true – Peter Florjančič notwithstanding.

There are a particular group of individuals who indeed are 'getting more', almost certainly, than you are. They are the same team who are likely to be getting more particularly during a lockdown or amid the social restrictions of a pandemic. In visitor numbers their bedrooms resemble Piccadilly Circus, partly because they are better at initiating conversation with prospective targets.

An essential reason we hold back from chatting up others is that we feel awkward and this is because we make assumptions about how others are negatively judging our social performance.

However, we are most likely to overcome our inhibitions when we get crazy with desire.

Eunsoo Choi of Georgetown University, USA, and Taekyun Hur[2] of Korea University examined whether confusion could originate from our strong tendency to 'project' – in other words, when we are 'up for it', we tend to assume the samer of others we encounter. Men may project onto women their own sexual interest, for instance.

As an example, Choi and Hur noted that previous research has found that men suffering unsatisfying sex were more likely to interpret women's behaviour as sexually suggestive compared with those enjoying better sex lives.

Choi and Hur's study found women's seduction approaches were only influenced by their own sexual motivation, and not by their perception of sexual intent in men. Women would initiate 'courtship' only when they themselves were sexually motivated. In contrast, even without initial high sexual motivation, male participants in the experiment increased courtship when they perceived sexual intention from the female target.

As women are 'sexual gatekeepers' they may be less influenced by how up for sex a man is, because it makes sense for them to remain choosy, no matter how much sexual interest they are receiving.

Optimal female sexual strategy is to refuse to be so influenced by a partner's sexual intention but to be in control of choosing the partner she desires. In contrast, men tend to feel more encouraged to approach a woman if they believe she is sending them what they perceive to be inviting signals.

The best sexual strategy for men is to focus on getting women interested, rather than just assuming that they are. Meanwhile women might consider that at least some men could be truly loyal.

Choi and Hur's study also found certain lures are particularly attractive.

Combatting loneliness is vital in tackling the inevitable social isolation of the pandemic; establishing contact with others becomes essential to survival. However, you don't need to be extravert or suave. To be effective, you just need to take certain positive steps. Many of them will feel awkward and clunky at the beginning, yet these are core ingredients of the mental vaccine. It is the belief that you have to be impossibly sexy or charming that defeats most; instead, you just need to do the simple things on this list. Some may not appear relevant if you are trapped in the middle of a lockdown, but they can be adapted to this predicament. Performing the tasks on this list will overcome the awkwardness of breaking down social barriers.

The top ten seduction strategies most likely to maximise interest as uncovered by this study are ranked below, in descending order of how attractive they were found:

(1) Pay attention and listen in an interested way
(2) Look often and smile
(3) Make a joke and begin a conversation
(4) Reduce distance and start to talk
(5) Look often in order to obtain eye contact
(6) Approach and sit next to
(7) Directly express interest and invite to dance (e.g. make a compliment, offer a drink, say directly what you think of them)
(8) Talk indirectly, apparently in a functional way (e.g. ask what time it is, ask for a light, etc.)
(9) Try to look as physically desirable as possible
(10) Approach through a friend or people around

Choi and Hur obtained their list from an original survey by Carolina de Weerth of the University of Groningen) and Akko Kalma[3] of the University of Utrecht in which 163 young people described eighty-four different ways of letting a person of the opposite gender know that they were interested.

Is the psychological paradox at the heart of desire that emotion clouds our ability to spot what's real, and what isn't, in love? And are there some people more skilled in love precisely because they deploy their intelligence rather than their emotions?

First there was academic IQ, which predicted exam performance; then came emotional intelligence, which explained general social success; now there is mating IQ or mating intelligence, which is the way academic psychologists refer to the ability to seduce.

Among the first psychologists to originate the concept, Daniel O'Brien, Glenn Geher and Scott Barry Kaufman were part of a larger team that published one of the first studies on mating IQ.[4] Scoring higher on seduction skills or mating intelligence involves reading the minds of those you are attracted to, and being better at assessing their interest.

Sexual harassment might therefore partly arise out of low mating IQ. A high mating IQ was also found to be linked to general confidence in one's attractiveness, as well as the ability to manipulate potential mates. Women superior on mating IQ score higher on 'commitment scepticism', which translates into being better at seeing through feigned interest in longer-term relationships.

The investigation found that men scoring higher on mating IQ had more hook-ups, defined as uncommitted sexual encounters between consenting parties ranging from simple kissing to 'heavy petting' and intercourse.

The study, entitled 'Self-Perceived Mating Intelligence Predicts Sexual Behaviour in College Students: Empirical Validation of a Theoretical Construct', argued that women use hook-ups as screening for potential long-term mates.

This would imply fewer hook-ups with unfamiliar strangers (most likely to desert or deliver other unwanted consequences, e.g. disease), and fewer hook-ups with close friends, since such friendships were not founded on developing a sexual connection. For women, these psychologists argued, the most promising choice for a hook-up is an acquaintance, as some prior connection provides an opportunity to judge trustworthiness.

Women with high mating IQ were more likely to engage in acquaintance hook-ups but not with strangers or friends. The psychologists also found that women who are more confident in their mating skills engaged in sex at an earlier age. Women seemed to manifest a higher or lower mating IQ earlier in life, while male mating IQ seemed to develop over a more extended period of time and age.

It could be that men take longer to develop the skills they need to flirt, such as how to hold more attractive conversations. Another possibility is the issue of sincerity – which may take more time to learn to fake.

In one of the largest studies of its kind ever published, US psychologists have found a particular aspect of personality in men and women that predicts what the researchers refer to as 'hypersexuality'.[5] The 'hypersexual' have more sexual partners than the rest of the population, fantasise more about people other than their current partner, and tend to favour more sex without love. They take greater pleasure in casual sex with different partners, and don't need attachment to enjoy lovemaking.

Hypersexuality was found strongly linked with a particular aspect of personality.

Another especially intriguing aspect of this research, conducted on 482 people aged between seventeen and fifty-six, was that this personality feature applied equally to both men and women in predicting hypersexuality. Psychologists are beginning to concur that it's this unique element of character which most powerfully predicts higher numbers of different sexual partners, as well as impulsive one-night stands, and a gamut of risky sexual behaviours.

This character trait is psychopathy.

Psychopaths are linked in the popular imagination with criminals and sex offenders, but psychologists Rebecca Kastner and Martin Sellbom[5] emphasise they were studying features of psychopathy which are more common in the general population than may be realised.[6]

Do we need to look closer to home, in this pandemic, for psychopathic tendencies in those who break COVID rules?

Other studies directly examining this issue found those reporting high levels of antisociality or psychopathy engage in fewer social distancing measures, leave their homes more frequently even in lockdown and stand closer to others while outside, while also exhibiting less attention to hygiene.

Psychopaths ignore restrictions on socialising during a pandemic and so they are going to be the ones most available for hook-ups during this time. But there is more.

Psychologists believe everyone falls somewhere along the spectrum of psychopathy, and have more or less of these traits. It would seem the more aspects of psychopathy are reflected in a person's character, the more they embrace 'hypersexuality'.

The psychopathic personality is characterised by a callous and manipulative approach to others, lack of remorse, plus deceit, all covered up by superficial charm. This is not a particularly alluring package at first glance, so psychologists have been probing deeper inside the psychopath's mind, unlocking the secret of their success in the bedroom.

Kastner and Sellbom found from their study that it's the 'Fearless-Dominance' aspect of psychopathy, combined with the 'Impulsive-Antisocial' element, which explains why psychopaths dominate the medal tables in the sexual Olympics.

Fearlessness and dominance means psychopaths appear charming, grandiose, risk-taking with little regard for consequences, combined with an absence of anxiety. They don't anticipate and aren't bothered by performance failure – which is a consideration that might put the rest of us off being hypersexual. These factors can also be positively associated with a good work ethic, even heroism, confidence and achievement – all characteristics that women value in a male partner.

Kastner and Sellbom also contend it's the relative immunity from stress and fearlessness of psychopaths which explains why they are less inhibited than the rest of us. As a result, they seek thrilling, dangerous, and otherwise anxiety-provoking sexual situations.

Psychologists argue it's the 'impulsive-antisocial' element of their character which ensures they use others ruthlessly for their own gain. This exploitative social style helps generate higher numbers of sexual partners and short-term mating. Impulsivity means they also act on possible rewards (like sex) without considering the consequences. They also disregard social norms and standards (one shall not be promiscuous, break the law, etc.).

One theory is that male and female psychopaths end up hypersexual through different routes via contrasts in personality – it's the antisocial aspect in men, but instead the impulsive thrill-seeking in women.

Psychologist David Kosson and colleagues[7] found in their research that of more psychopathic individuals, 58 per cent report using flattery, 40 per cent argument and 40 per cent exploitation of an intoxicated person to achieve sex. The figures from this study, entitled 'Psychopathy-Related Traits Predict Self-Reported Sexual Aggression Among College Men', and published in the *Journal of Interpersonal Violence*, were about twice as high as in the non-psychopathic.

Luna Muñoz and colleagues[8] researched sexually coercive tactics after being turned down by a partner, including sexual arousal and touching, emotional manipulation, exploiting by intoxication and physical force. The study found men and women rated high on psychopathy were more likely to be sexually coercive.

Based on her clinical experience, Dr Helinä Häkkänen-Nyholm,[9] a former criminal profiler of the Finnish police, found psychopathic women are more likely than others to engage in sexual coercion when they encounter conflict in their relationship. Clashes, in their minds, are solved by sex. Perhaps psychopathic women view sex as a tool for manipulating others and achieving what they want, whilst psychopathic men favour deceitful emotional engagement.

One of Dr Helinä Häkkänen-Nyholm's clients described (she reports this with his permission) an attempt to leave the marital home after announcing his intention to divorce, following years of mistreatment, betrayal and abuse. While standing in the corridor, he witnessed his wife undressing and suggesting sex.

Research has found psychopaths are also more interested in violent, coercive and sadistic sex, so this insight might unlock one of the secrets to the success of the best-selling novel *Fifty Shades of Grey*, where sado-masochistic coupling is part of the appeal of this publishing phenomenon.

This latest study reveals that any medal-winning sexual athlete has to be more psychopathic than we had realised before. So does *Fifty Shades of Grey* expose that deep in the recesses of all our personalities there lurks a sneaking admiration for psychopathic success in the bedroom?

Another predictor of how active your sex life is has been found to be your tendency to feel the emotion of disgust. Returning back to the toilet paper tissue at issue in Chapter 8, there is another link with disgust and how likely you are to be engage in sexual activities during the pandemic or lockdown.

Your proneness to feeling disgusted in everyday life also predicts elevated coronavirus anxiety and 'safety behaviours' during the pandemic.[10] Safety behaviour refers to avoidance of contamination, excessive washing or even overuse of medical supplies. The tendency to feel disgust plays a strong role in avoiding disease transmission.

Academics at Northern Illinois University point out[11] that to have sex, we have to overcome strong feelings of disgust.

Their study was partly inspired by the observation that the human body is pretty disgusting. It secretes fluids and harbours germs, and we generally find contact with anything that has been in a stranger's body extremely unpleasant. The genitals and mouth are involved in sex, yet are also the regions that might be associated with most disgust. Despite all that possible repulsion in reaction to such orifices and secretions, we still make love.

The authors point out that the act of physical intimacy presents us with an evolutionary dilemma: we want to avoid contamination from potentially dangerous substances, and yet we are also motivated to attain mates, as we do need to pass on our genes.

Ellen Lee, James Ambler and Brad Sagarin[11] suggest a possible way nature has resolved this dilemma: an internal mechanism that evolved in our brains inhibiting disgust in 'reproductively-relevant situations'.

This means that sexual arousal reduces revulsion.

The study found that in women, sexual arousal significantly lowered sexual disgust. The authors argue that their findings support the evolutionary theory that erotic arousal inhibits distaste, which facilitates a willingness to engage in high-risk, but evolutionarily necessary, procreation.

The authors also argue that this effect could be particularly important for women.

In this research men showed very low levels of sexual disgust, even when not sexually aroused, indicating a potential 'floor effect' – in other words, the measured repugnance was so small in the first place that it had nowhere to go in terms of getting lower with sexual arousal. Research has found women more sensitive than men to revulsion, particularly to sexual disgust.

However, the authors also point out that the item on the sexual disgust subscale that showed the least decrease in revulsion with arousal was sexual attention from a disliked source: 'Finding out that someone you don't like has sexual fantasies about you.' Being turned on does not appear to make unwanted sexual attention or partners more palatable, particularly in women.

A study entitled 'Disgust and mating strategy'[12] has found that our feelings and attitudes to disgust could also be part of our personality, and in particular are linked to mating, love or sex strategies.

The study started from the fact that people generally vary in their attitudes and desire for longer-term, committed relationships versus short-term, uncommitted connections. It follows we should also expect those who are more inclined toward 'short-term mating' to experience lower levels of sexual disgust.

The authors point out successful short-term mating strategies typically involve multiple sexual partners, desire for sexual variety, and brief intervals of time between meeting and sexual intercourse.

This strategy should be difficult to implement in the presence of high levels of sexual disgust. Those with higher levels of such repulsion are less likely to be comfortable with casual sex, multiple partners and sex that occurs before sufficient information can be acquired about the health and hygiene status of potential mates.

The authors, therefore, propose that a crucial component of a successful short-term mating strategy is lower sexual disgust. In contrast, reduced repulsion regarding certain aspects of sex is not necessary for the successful pursuit of a more monogamous strategy.

One possible speculation from these new findings is that higher levels of sexual disgust may even facilitate the implementation of committed mating strategies by inhibiting short-term mating and deterring those in committed relationships from sexual infidelity.

The research asked participants to rate how disgusting they find a variety of potentially repellent situations, for example 'a stranger of the opposite sex intentionally rubbing your thigh in an elevator' and 'performing oral sex'.

The study found that a stronger disposition toward short-term mating is associated with reduced sexual disgust.

The investigation also found that the relationship between physical attractiveness and short-term mating was significantly stronger in men. More physically attractive men are keener on short-term flings, while more physically attractive women are not more interested in such an approach to their sex lives.

The authors argue that physically attractive women may have a larger number of sexual partners simply because they have more eager suitors, or have sex at an earlier age, but not necessarily because they are pursuing a 'short-term mating strategy'. Women's attractiveness in this research was not associated with desire for, or positive attitudes toward, short-term mating.

The authors argue that shorter-term mating looms larger in men's than in women's relationship psychology, and is pursued more vigorously by men because as a strategy it has evolutionary benefits for men, in terms of passing on more genes.

This pattern is apparently mirrored in other species: more attractive male birds devote less effort to parenting when they can translate their physical attractiveness into 'extra-pair copulations'.

Maybe the quality of your sex life generally can be predicted by levels of disgust.[13]

Might this new research possibly also suggest an intriguing new way of predicting how likely your partner is to stay or stray? Perhaps we can analyse them by how disgusted they are by certain aspects of intimacy, or how rapidly their levels of disgust vanish as they get turned on?

Maybe the next time you are on a date and trying to work out if the relationship has a future, you should produce the bucket used in that Freudian 'anal personality type' study...

11

LONELINESS UNDER LOCKDOWN

Does the film The Full Monty *lay bare the secret solution to solitude? Is there a link with pop star Beyoncé's bare-faced cheek?*

Could one of the secrets of staying alive during the pandemic be revealed by pop star Beyoncé?[1]

The Scottish government[2] has declared on its website that over 80 per cent of people in Scotland have felt awkward when trying to follow the new social distancing or mask wearing rules. A majority have been concerned about appearing rude or hurting someone's feelings.

It is this awkwardness which could prevent you from properly protecting yourself from Covid. If you don't overcome feeling embarrassed, and instead act assertively in the face of others who are invading your personal space in a dangerous manner, then it will be awkwardness that ends up doing you in, not the virus.[2]

Overcoming awkwardness also lies at the centre of the issue of breaking down the various barriers involving shyness and fears of rejection which stop you making more connections with others.

How will Beyoncé help you?

A television audience of millions watched President Barack Obama get sworn in for his second term in office on 21 January 2013, a glittering ceremony which included performances by elite stars who should have been at top of their game, including James Taylor, Kelly Clarkson and Beyoncé.[1]

But following her performance of the Star-Spangled Banner, doubts later emerged over whether Beyoncé had in fact recorded her vocal as opposed to genuinely performing live. This rapidly turned into a kind of scandal, being stoked by social media speculation and mounting press coverage of the issue.

Beyoncé is usually referred to purely by her first name but her full name is Beyoncé Giselle Knowles-Carter. The diva later confirmed that she had indeed mimed her performance, but perhaps somewhat defensively she explained she's a 'perfectionist' and – due to lack of rehearsal time – 'did not feel comfortable taking a risk'.

'I wanted to make him [Obama] and my country proud, so I decided to sing along with my pre-recorded track ... I'm very proud of my performance,' she said. As long as this defence continued, it might appear she was digging a hole for herself, but luckily, she quickly abandoned that strategy and came up with an altogether much more effective one.

It is a tactic we can all learn from.

To make a point, Beyoncé opened the press conference where she was supposed to answer these allegations by asking reporters to stand, before giving a rousing rendition of the national anthem.

Only after she had turned in a stunning acapella performance did she turn to the assembled press pack and ask, 'Any questions?'

Who was going to dare to interrogate her singing ability after that?

But many will still be wondering if she just got a bit nervous at the inauguration, or whether this shows how self-doubt can creep into the minds of even the most ostentatiously confident performers. No one, it seems, dared to say directly to her, if you can sing like that at the press conference, why didn't you just do that at the inauguration?

Nervousness can afflict even the most seasoned performer so the fear of being judged negatively by others is so common as to be ... pandemic.

The 1997 BAFTA-winning movie *The Full Monty* recounts how a group of unemployed steel workers reluctantly resolve to form a male striptease act. They're forced to strip in order to survive financially; Sheffield has been denuded of the industrial jobs that are their lifeblood.

While appearing on a TV chat show programme discussing the backstory to *The Full Monty* a while ago, I was privileged enough to meet some real-life male characters who had gone down this route due to financial pressure, remarkably similar to the film plot. I wasn't there in my capacity as a fellow stripper. Instead, I was asked to discuss the psychology of the predicament of baring all, for the first time, in front of strangers when it's not your chosen career.

It was fascinating to see psychological theory in action in the real world. Precisely vindicating what neuroscience would predict, these men, who had no history of being performers on stage, were indeed mortified with their first few uncoordinated attempts. However, as time passed, they became gradually more attuned to the demands of the situation, until, just as the behavioural science would anticipate, they, to a man, eventually became blasé about strutting their stuff stark naked in front of a room full of screaming women.

What on earth has any of this got to do with overcoming loneliness under lockdown? What is the link with overcoming the awkwardness of initiating a social encounter, which is indeed the same psychology as overpowering the fear of annoying someone by asking them to keep two metres away?

Accounts from the actors in the actual movie indicate that the shooting of one scene did require them to disrobe fully, for a rowdy female crowd. This in the end was only facilitated through the imbibing of alcohol. Even experienced actors, it seems, needed 'Dutch courage'.

The theme here is the notion of awkwardness. This is one of the central predicaments the isolated must overcome if they are to initiate contact with others. Those who end up lonely also tend to harbour stronger feelings of social clumsiness, and this inhibits them from taking the plunge, initiating conversations.

When faced with awkward predicaments, like initiating contact with strangers or starting heart-to-hearts or breaking down barriers of lonesomeness, you will need to overcome strong feelings of social ineptitude.

Feeling gauche or gawky is extremely common and is one of the basic barriers to being assertive about social isolation, as well as confronting people when they are not observing the new rules of social distancing or wearing face masks and so exposing you to risk.

On 7 December 2020 the Scottish government published on their website 'Coronavirus (COVID-19): dealing with awkward social situations – guidance'. The subtitle was: 'Information to support anyone who may struggle with challenging or awkward social situations when interacting with other people under the current coronavirus restrictions'.[2]

'A friend goes in for a hug or handshake' was the first predicament; the official advice: *Changing how we say hello to one another isn't easy. Being honest about it can make things easier.*

They recommend the following: 'I so want to hug you! But I guess we have to wait until it's safe. I don't want to risk harming you or anyone else you are in contact with. I'm giving you a virtual hug.'

This is not such bad advice, but it doesn't help people by giving them the foundation on which it is based so that they can take away the guiding principles to use in whatever particular gawky encounter they experience.

One principle perhaps so obvious that it got overlooked by the Scottish government is that in order to escape from these new and various social predicaments, you are going to have to resort to telling little stories which are not exactly lies, but which are intended to ensure you get your way without hurting the feelings of others. This 'game playing' is an essential social survival skill, particularly in situations where you are unlikely to have to endure continuing intimacy over an extended period (when brutal honesty is more sustainable in the longer term).

One key principle is to always frame the response in terms of a question. This achieves several very powerful psychological ends. Queries naturally take control of a conversation as there is a powerful human tendency to respond by diverting attention and intellectual resources to answering questions.

Questions tend to put the ball back into the court of the other person and turn the awkwardness back at them. Later in this chapter we are going to see from some psychological research how certain questions are most powerful in terms of flirting and seducing, but the key principle that applies here, as in other predicaments in life, is that it all boils down to asking the right question.

A better response to the Scottish government's scenario, in my opinion, might be to keep most of what they suggested but change the bit about waiting until it's safe to: 'What are your thoughts about waiting until its actually safe?' There are ways of framing questions so that it would be very difficult for anyone to disagree, and this is a powerful mental technique for engineering the outcome you want.

This is clearly a highly manipulative strategy, and is about another key point the government advice doesn't clarify: you need to be clear with yourself about your goal, and that you are happy to use whatever manipulative techniques necessary to get others to bend to your will.

Scenario number 2 on the Scottish Government website:[2] 'Someone you know removes their mask indoors'. Their advice is: *You've seen a colleague in a coffee shop and they take off their mask to speak to you. Always assume that people have the best intentions, and that they may have forgotten or misunderstood the current guidance. In this situation, you could offer an explanation and an alternative. 'Let's catch up outside? Where there's space to keep a wee distance.'*

The problem with this advice is that there is a danger of it being misinterpreted that you are unhappy being too close to the friend for other reasons. A better way of getting outside is to suggest it for reasons that are unambiguous and maybe that means you don't mention the health guidelines. I prefer: *'Is it me or is it getting rather stuffy in here, would you mind if we stepped outside as I am finding it difficult to breathe in here!'*

In my opinion this is a superior tactic, although more manipulative because you are not being strictly honest about why you want to step outside. However, you are more likely to get an affirmative, because the way you have framed the question makes it very difficult for anyone to disagree. Notice that even the Scottish government doesn't advise directly confronting your colleague over the fact they took off their face mask.

According to the Scottish Government: *The rules are there to protect us all so if the person becomes confrontational it's OK to report it to the nearest staff member.* In these and other example responses they seem rather trigger-happy on 'report to the authorities if necessary' type responses. This is very unlikely to leave you with much of a social life if you keep following their advice and report all and sundry to those in charge.

At least the Scottish government has at some level acknowledged that part of the huge new stress of the pandemic is how to negotiate new rules and new kinds of relationships within those unusual predicaments. The idea that there is inevitably going to be awkwardness needs to be more embraced, however.

At the deepest level of facing up to the predicament of feeling mortified when you reach out to others, if you want the gold medal in the social skills Olympics, as you feel ashamed, you really need to lean into the awkwardness.

Careening into the cringe relates to this essential idea of tolerating your own vulnerability. If you can stand to be seen to be imperfect, that gives you power. You could, at the most powerful level of all, explain that you are feeling awkward. Over and over again it turns out we warm to those who are honest about feeling maladroit, rather than rejecting them.

Those who consider themselves socially unpolished need to abandon the idea that their goal is to aim for deft social performance and instead embrace their floundering, perhaps even drawing attention to it. The shy harbour unrealistic standards over how witty and self-assured everyone else is, comparing their own ineptness unfavourably.

We're often intimidated by those in conversation who seem to know more, and indeed seem to apprehend everything, and can declaim on any subject with an intelligent and forthright opinion. But in fact, the truly intellectually respectable response is – far from attempting to bluff your way through – to own up to your ignorance, and declare, 'I don't get it. Explain it to me.'

You can only lean into your awkwardness if you also believe, as outlined above, that while things may be tough to begin with, in the long run you'll overcome resistance and the others will warm to you.

In an experiment[3] involving mock-job interviews, an interviewee was in a wheelchair, either acknowledging or not acknowledging the possible stigma that might interfere with getting hired. 'Acknowledgement' as a tactic in this case took the form of the statement, 'When people meet me, one of the first things that they notice is that I use a wheelchair.'

There is a sense in which this statement directly confronts and acknowledges the awkwardness which might have enveloped the situation, but has remained unsaid. Obviously, no one involved in this research is arguing that the wheelchair should in any sense prevent someone from being hired, but if it is causing awkwardness, even if it shouldn't, it might be more powerful psychologically to put the issue front and centre, rather than avoid it.

The experiment found individuals who may be facing prejudice against them, particularly perhaps if the bias remained unsaid, were more likely to be hired when they acknowledged their obvious difference.

'Acknowledgement' as a tactic in these experiments was achieved by altering the response to a question regarding why the applicant should be hired. One group of applicants 'acknowledged' their physical appearance by saying in the application, 'I know that I don't look like your typical construction worker, but...' Elsewhere in the application another statement was inserted to the effect: 'I know that there are not a lot of ... in this industry, but...'

This notion of the self-fulfilling prophecy is vital in the next step to battling social isolation. People end up alone because they believe they will be rejected if they try to reach out to others. Those who are convinced that, no matter what resistance they initially meet, they will eventually be socially successful and so persist *are* indeed successful. The impact of the self-fulfilling prophecy, particularly when it comes to initiating conversations with strangers, has been startlingly demonstrated in one of the most famous experiments in social psychology.

The power of expectation was examined in a 1977 study[4] by a team led by Mark Snyder in which men were shown photographs of a woman to whom they would be talking by phone. The woman in the pictures was randomised to being either extremely physically attractive or unattractive (as rated by other independent observers).

What the men taking part in the experiment didn't know was that those sneaky psychologists had told a porky pie, and the photographs were not only randomly assigned to the men, but they also did not correspond in any way to the actual woman with whom they had the phone conversation.

While it would come as no surprise that the men behaved differently to the women during the phone conversation depending on their (manipulated) beliefs regarding her physical appearance, the really surprising finding was that independent ratings of the women's segments of the conversations revealed that females whose conversational partners believed them to be less appealing behaved in a less attractive fashion (i.e. they were rated as sounding less warm and interesting).

The women had also been kept completely in the dark by the psychologists about the photograph manipulation. They were not aware it had taken place. This effect, therefore, had to have been mediated in some way through the men's behaviour. One possibility is that the men who were talking to someone they believed to be unattractive were less affable than men who believed they were talking to an attractive woman. This in turn had an impact on the way the women responded, and the way they then subsequently came over to an independent observer.

A version of this powerful effect of expectation is known within academic psychology as the Pygmalion Effect. In ancient Greek mythology, Pygmalion, King of Cyprus, sculpted a beautiful feminine form 'out of ivory and desire', named it Galatea and promptly fell in love with it. The power of his relentless desire, combined with assistance from the goddess Aphrodite, transformed the statue into a living woman.

The Pygmalion Effect is a special instance of the self-fulfilling prophecy where having an expectation of another causes the interlocutor to modify their performance so it falls into line with the expectation of the first party.

Dorsha Hayes[5] explains in a paper entitled 'The Archetypal Nature of Stage Fright' that this mysterious condition is best understood from the standpoint of a person as a part of a herd, attached to the primary safety of the pack. To make oneself conspicuous is, in her analysis, to detach oneself from the pack. Historically, separation from the group has always been precarious. These fears are deeply embedded below conscious awareness, she argues; and being before an audience may induce this primitive fear to erupt from our archetypal memory.

Her paper contends that standing alone is to be vulnerable and helpless against massed attack. Facing an audience reminds our brains at a primitive level of this confrontation. It was the outcast, the victim, the tortured, the stoned to death and the crucified who, through history, faced the crowd.

While she might have a point, the treatment of social phobia, public speaking fears and stage fright is an action-oriented therapy, which means to get out there, in a graded manner, and do it, not to avoid it; but on the other hand also to regulate breathing throughout the experience.

Notwithstanding the question of whether there is an archetypal primitive memory or not, we can learn to become comfortable before spectators if given enough exposure, in a graded manner, by slowly increasing the size of the audience we are exposed to.

We don't know if Beyoncé had stage fright or not, but choosing to sing at the press conference was the correct cure, and a great idea. There is a sense in which singing before taking questions directly confronted the awkwardness at the heart of her predicament. She could have chosen to defend her position over miming with a host of defensive arguments. Instead, she belted out the song at the press conference afterwards, slaying any questions over her ability to sing. She turned the situation around by asking the assembled press pack if they had any questions, which now seemed a bit redundant as she had answered any possible question over her singing ability and her nerves by delivering a stand-out performance at the press conference convened to question what happened at the inauguration ceremony.

If we want to tackle loneliness related to feelings of awkwardness over pandemic restrictions, or at any time, the research tells us: in any awkward situation take the bull by the horns and act. *Confront* rather than running and hiding.

And there is more subtle guidance from psychology studies, drilling down further into making good conversation. The secret to attractive conversations was recently uncovered by a psychology study entitled 'It Doesn't Hurt to Ask: Question-asking increases Liking'.

A team of psychologists led by Karen Huang and Francesca Gino[6] found people who asked a higher rate of a very specific type of question in conversation were more liked, and were asked on more second dates. Studies of conversations in public settings such as bars and trains have found that two-thirds of conversations are spent talking about personal experiences, but also that focusing on yourself decreases your appeal. The authors argue that asking questions increases liking because it indicates responsiveness, which can be further divided as demonstrating three crucial components everyone is looking for: understanding, validation and care.

By asking questions, you acknowledge that the partner's perspective is valuable enough that you want to know more. The authors of the study classified the standard question types that occur in conversation.

The different types of question are 'follow-up', where the question naturally follows on from what the other person has just said and is a further inquiry into their experience; 'full switch', a complete, perhaps abrupt, change of subject; 'partial switch', a question that seems related to what came before but is also moving the person away from what they were just talking about; 'mirror', where you ask something very closely linked to what you have just been asked; 'introductory', a standard opening question to get the conversation going; and 'rhetorical', when something more abstract is probed and not usually related to an immediate experience being discussed.

This study found that it is follow-up questions which hit the flirting jackpot and are particularly likely to increase liking. This is because they most represent responsiveness from the questioner. Neglecting to ask questions altogether may reveal you are egocentric, focused on expressing your own thoughts, feelings and beliefs with little or no interest in hearing what another has to say – an ominous sign when it comes to flirting.

Here are some examples of questions from Huang and Gino's study:

Follow-up (this one is best for flirting)
'I'm planning a trip to Canada.'
Question: 'Oh, cool. Have you ever been there before?'

Full switch
'I am working at a dry-cleaners.'
Question: 'What do you like doing for fun?'

Partial switch
'Not super outdoorsy, but not opposed to a hike or something once in a while.'
Question: 'Have you been to the beach much in Boston?'

Mirror
'What did you have for breakfast?
Question: 'I had eggs and fruit. How about you?'

Introductory
'Hello!'
Question: 'Hey, how's it going?'

Rhetorical
'What's the craziest event you've been to?'
Question: 'Yesterday I followed a marching band around. Where were they going? It's a mystery.'

The power of this way of categorising conversation is that it allows participants to become more aware of what their options are at any one moment in any dialogue. This is a massive boost in becoming more skilled. It also helps you observe more clearly what others are doing, as you can label each technique as you recognise it being deployed.

There is no mysterious 'x-factor' or secret ingredient to great conversation, but there are rules. Anyone can follow them and use them to their advantage. However, no matter how skilled you become, it is inevitable you are still going to put your foot in it, and need to apologise afterwards, and confront the inevitable awkwardness. It is part of the human predicament.

Frank Fincham published a paper entitled 'The kiss of the porcupines: from attributing responsibility to forgiving',[7] which argued that the human condition is a bit like two porcupines kissing: the way we invariably dig into each other means that forgiveness and apology are central to relationships.

Fincham asks us to imagine two porcupines huddled together in the cold of an Alaskan winter's night, each providing life-sustaining warmth to the other. As the porcupines draw closer together, the painful pricks from each other's quills repel them. But then the need for warmth brings them together again.

This 'kiss of the porcupines' is a metaphor for the human condition. Humans harm each other and yet we are also social animals. The paper, published in the academic journal *Personal Relationships*, explains that the 'kiss of the porcupines' is about how to relate to others in the face of the inevitable hazards of being harmed.

Fincham points out that in close relationships we voluntarily make ourselves defenceless. Rendering ourselves vulnerable is a double-edged sword. It makes possible the profound sense of security that can be experienced in close relationships. At the same time, the flaws of any partner mean that hurt or injury is inevitable. The wound is particularly distressing precisely because we have emotionally exposed ourselves.

12

THE GOOD FEUD GUIDE

How to win any argument germane to the germ

The pandemic has presented us with a huge quantity of quandaries, upon which we don't all seem able to agree. It ends up feeling like we're in the middle of incessant divisive national referenda on problems about which people are passionate but can't ever seem to settle.

It's a bit like Brexit in how it constantly appears to divide us irreconcilably. Should schools be open? Should you send your child to school? Should you wear a face mask? Should there be a lockdown? Should the government provide financial support, and, if so, how much? Should you be standing quite so close? Best friends end up quarrelling about quarantine, while siblings squabble about social distancing – and so it goes on.

It turns out that Brexit was bad for your mental health. If this is the case then it follows the divisiveness of lockdown will probably have just as severe an effect, if not worse.

According to a study conducted by a psychologist at Bangor University, outnumbered Brexiteers living in Remain-voting areas suffer poorer mental health than their pro-EU neighbours, while 'remainers' living in Leave-voting areas also had worse mental health than their Brexit-voting neighbours in the same way.

Dr Chris Saville[1] contends that the 2016 referendum created new minority groups, and that the resulting polarised politics had a significant public health impact:

A few years ago, the idea that someone's opinions on EU membership not matching that of their neighbours could be bad for their mental health would be ridiculous. It's a real demonstration of just how quickly social identities form and how powerful they can be.

The study, entitled 'Mental health consequences of minority political positions: the case of Brexit' confirms that finding yourself part of a minority group, even one that has developed quickly because of a very recent shift in political circumstance, could negatively affect your mental health.

It would appear the same could be said of the pandemic and the splitting over government policies such as social distancing, lockdowns and wearing face masks. This argumentative divisiveness, as we have seen, has deep implications for our well-being in the midst of all the other strains. Constant fruitless arguing can leave us just as frazzled as any of the other hits from the current horror.

This is not a guide on what the right answers are. Instead, it is an analysis of the psychology of how to have an argument and how to settle one in the midst of irreconcilable differences. This is vital if we are to move beyond the divisiveness.

Let us examine how professional debaters win. What could you learn from the best politicians on how to defeat your opponent in a battle of wills and wits? Could it help you end all those tiffs over transmission?

This notion of interruption, as we shall see, appears to have become central to how modern-day arguments are won or lost in the highest-stakes arena of all: politicians feuding on TV. Perhaps the most successful politician of the TV age in the last century was the UK's Margaret Thatcher, who – whether you agreed with her politics or not – appeared streets ahead of her adversaries of the day in rhetorical skill.

Psychologists Peter Bull and Kate Mayer[2] analysed in unparalleled depth Prime Minister Thatcher's performances in TV interviews. Their analysis reveals that she deployed psychological techniques which appear to have given her a crucial edge.

In their study, eight televised interviews were selected from four different interviewers, who each interrogated both Margaret Thatcher and then Leader of the Opposition Neil Kinnock, and the video recordings were analysed. The interviews analysed were conducted by Sir Robin Day, Jonathan Dimbleby, David Dimbleby and David Frost.

No significant difference was found between Margaret Thatcher and Neil Kinnock either in the extent to which they interrupted, or were interrupted by, the interviewers. Where the politicians did diverge was in the degree to which they explicitly protested at being interrupted. Thatcher objected to being interrupted much more than Kinnock did.

The psychologists contend that this gave the misleading impression that she was being excessively interrupted, although the objective evidence uncovered in the study clearly shows a striking similarity in both the frequency and pattern of interruptions between the two politicians.

The impression created by this psychological device is that she was badly treated.

On one occasion investigated in this study, Jonathan Dimbleby was reduced to apologising for asking questions. The psychologists conclude that Margaret Thatcher revealed a striking mastery of the arts of political one-upmanship, continually wrong-footing interviewers and putting them on the defensive, such that they felt obliged to justify and even apologise for their role as interviewers.

Margaret Thatcher's death has provoked heated controversy over her legacy. Behavioural scientists have uncovered evidence suggesting she was an outstanding proponent of psychologically manipulative techniques. Perhaps, among other things, she ushered in a new era of ultra-wily political strategy on TV.

This has led over the years to the inevitable present-day outcome: that the microphones of the candidates in the final Trump-Biden Presidential Debate were switched off, preventing interruptions by either party, for at least part of the televised encounter.

This follows widespread negative reaction from the audience to the extensive interposing that characterised the first verbal TV tussle. But as these two adversaries are experienced campaigners, does there continue to be a hidden, ever-developing powerful psychology behind the tactic of interjecting?

Could you use this to your advantage when trying to achieve more dominance and assertiveness? The very fact that a technological solution had to be sought suggests this conversational tactic might be a more powerful weapon than is commonly realised. Political and psychological strategists behind the scenes and behind both candidates may be increasingly advocating interruption as a rhetorical weapon.

What do they know that we don't?

Research by psychologists conducting scientific experiments on the impact of interrupting find that those who interrupt more are indeed evaluated as more capable, confident, dominant and persuasive. But this comes at a price: they are also usually seen as less likeable and attractive.[3]

Maybe in the middle of a pandemic voters are looking for the more dominant candidate and care less about how likeable they are?

The psychological consequences of interruption can be both positive (being seen as more assertive) yet also negative (coming over as rude). Interestingly this has been found to be especially true for female interrupters.[4]

Some of the research into interrupting has found that men interrupt (especially where it is intrusive interruption) more than women; concomitantly, women are more often interrupted than men are, and men interrupt women significantly more than they do other men.[5]

A lot depends on the precise kind of interruption and the timing; some wait for what looks like an approach to an ending before interrupting, while others leap in right at the start of a conversation.

Differing types of interruption with different effects include deep and 'intrusive' interruptions, which try to change the subject, and prevent the other person from speaking. However, there are also so-called 'overlapping interruptions', where a person appears to be coming to the end of making a point and the other person interrupts just before what would seem to be the natural end-point.

There are even so-called 'silent' interruptions where, for example, someone momentarily forgets the word they were looking for, or pauses to find the right phrase, and their adversary steps in to supply the correct word, yet then takes over the conversation.

A recent psychological experiment[6] investigating the effects of different kinds of interruption found, surprisingly, that so-called 'disagreement' interruptions (perhaps the kind that were most on display between Trump and Biden) were evaluated more positively by an audience than 'change-subject' interruptions. This positive evaluation did not disappear with high-frequency interruptions.

One theory the authors had for why 'disagreement' interruptions didn't suffer the same negative reception as 'change-subject' was that perhaps these interruptions at least suggested a strong engagement with the issue. It did not necessarily imply the same disregard for the speaker being interrupted as would have been the case if the interruption was 'change-subject'.

In other words, there appear to be ways of interrupting which look like they are justified because of passionate engagement with the issue. However, as a debating tactic where the aim is to defeat an opponent in rhetoric, interrupting has some powerful hidden psychology behind it.

For example, if you are aware that your opponent tends to interrupt and is constantly looking for an opportunity to 'take the floor' from you, then this may encourage you to speak faster than you normally would. The fear of providing an opportunity for the so-called 'silent' interruption may push you into unfamiliar conversational territory. In trying to prevent an interruption, you may not speak slowly or carefully or clearly enough... and thus stumble or misspeak, producing a verbal error your opponent can seize upon.

Also, if you are aware that your opponent is interrupting you and gaining more 'floor time' from you, then you may feel pressured into interrupting *them*; but if you are less skilled at this tactic then your timing may be poorer and your choice of opportunity may then reflect badly on you. You end up being the one coming over as rude.

There is even the tactic of interrupting by saying that you agree, which causes such surprise that the other speaker pauses and you seize the opportunity to explain that what you agreed with was not what they were hoping. For them not to allow you the chance to speak when you assert that you agree now makes them appear the ones seeking conflict and confrontation.

It could be that the real psychological power of interrupting isn't even on display in the speeches, but instead it disrupts thought patterns... and it is here that the real danger lies: it stops you thinking clearly, and thus insidiously achieves victory.

There is, however, another subtle and perhaps deeper aspect of interrupting. It establishes a power relationship between two people in a dialogue, perhaps even at an unconscious level.

It is well known that superiors in a hierarchy, say at the office, tend to interrupt underlings more than vice versa. It may be that some people, particularly those most interested in power, observe levels of interruption to identify whom they can and cannot dominate.

Researchers have found[7] that so-called 'sub-clinical' psychopaths (perhaps people who run offices rather than hold up banks) tended to detect who interrupted them more, and as a result, appeared to become less interested in a potentially exploitative future relationship. In other words, if you interrupt a psychopath while they try to make their point more than they are used to, they detect this quickly and they infer they may be less able to manipulate or use you, and they move on to other targets.

When Biden and Trump started interrupting each other, there was a lot more going on beneath the surface than just simple rudeness.

Arguing might be seen, in general, as an unpleasant activity which should be avoided at all costs in 'normal', everyday relationships. Politicians argue because they have opponents who must be defeated in order to gain power. They therefore resort to ever more wily strategies in order to win. But surely in everyday life, as opposed to political debates, arguing just creates opponents, and having lots of adversaries is not conducive to a happy life?

This is a question which has been investigated by a large psychological study entitled 'Some key differences between a happy life and a meaningful life',[8] published in the *Journal of Positive Psychology*.

How argumentative you were became a surprisingly important factor in determining how happy you were, and how pleasant you found life. The drive to argue, given it often led to less happiness, was about the pursuit of the *meaningful* life. That is fine; just realise that you are sacrificing happiness for meaning. And conversely, many forfeit meaning in life for happiness.

The researchers let participants define the happy, or meaningful life. Happiness appeared linked to having needs and desires satisfied, and leading an existence largely free from unpleasant events. A meaningful life, in contrast, appeared linked to some over-arching purpose. Often it meant sacrifice and being devoted to improving the welfare of others, rather than to yourself.

Attaining the 'holy grail' of the happy *and* meaningful life appeared possible from the findings of this study, but it is not as straightforward as previously might have been thought. Happiness flows from benefits you receive from others. Meaningfulness, on the other hand, is associated with the gains that others receive from you.

This new psychological research finds that while being happy and finding life meaningful overlap, there are important differences. A survey of 397 adults revealed that satisfying one's needs and wants increased happiness but was largely irrelevant to meaningfulness.

Happiness was linked to being a taker rather than a giver, whereas meaningfulness went more with being a giver rather than a taker. Higher levels of worry, stress and anxiety were linked to more meaningfulness, less happiness.

It might come as no surprise that the results reveal finding one's life to be relatively easy was linked to more happiness. But considering life a struggle was positively correlated with meaningfulness. Some people endure highly meaningful yet rather unpleasant lives, perhaps because their meaningful activities require strenuous and draining effort.

The authors, from Florida State University, Stanford University and the University of Minnesota, conclude that finding one's life easy or difficult is a matter of happiness, but not of meaning. The more time people devoted to thinking about the past and future, the more meaningful their lives were – and the less happy. Thinking beyond the present moment into the past or future was a sign of the relatively meaningful but unhappy life. The more people thought only about the present, the happier they were.

We first raised this vital issue when we discussed the need to find a place of safety, and how that might be the *present* when the future became scary, as it does in a pandemic.

Also, very relevant to travel and socialising restrictions during an epidemic is deciding whom to include in your social circle if you have to become brutally selective.

This study found that spending time with friends was positively related to happiness. Time spent with loved ones was significantly linked with meaning, but surprisingly irrelevant to happiness, possibly because loved ones can be difficult at times. People with more meaningful lives also agreed that 'relationships are more important than achievements'; this sentiment was unrelated to happiness.

For parents, the more time they spent taking care of children, the more meaningful their lives were; yet looking after children also reduced happiness. Becoming a parent has been shown by a raft of research often to reduce happiness. Roy Baumeister, the lead author of the study, has proposed that the 'parenthood paradox' can be resolved by proposing that we seek not just happiness but also meaning. People become parents because the gains in meaningfulness offset any losses in happiness.

This latest research by Roy Baumeister, Kathleen Vohs, Jennifer Aaker and Emily Garbinsky[8] has profound implications for positive psychology, because it suggests that people will pursue *meaningfulness* even at the expense of happiness.

In their study, the more that people regarded arguing as something that reflects *them* and their true inner self, the more meaningful but the less happy their lives were. The effects of arguing were similar, in this respect, to those of helping others.

The authors of the study propose that meaningfulness comes in part from being involved in things one regards as important, and sometimes one has to argue for these. But the unpleasantness of arguing may contribute to lower happiness. Happy people may prefer not to argue and arguing is something they might do only reluctantly, rather than as a frequent expression of their inner self and values.

It's again perhaps not surprising that more worrying was linked to less happiness, but that it was also associated with higher levels of meaningfulness. People with very meaningful lives worry more and have more stress than people with less meaningful lives.

The authors suggest that worrying comes from involvement and engagement with important activities that go beyond the self and the present, and so it may often be an unavoidable part of a meaningful life, even though it detracts from happiness.

What is the deeper insight within this research, when we feel the need to argue?

This study indicates that arguing can test our connections with others to destruction so should be done with caution. The more that people regarded arguing as something that reflected them, the more meaningful but less happy their lives were. Argument may be necessary in order to express your sense of who you are, your identity. Sometimes suppressing opposition buys you friendship but at the expense of really being you.

At some level most of our arguments are internal ones, where we argue with ourselves. In particular, we argue with ourselves over unpleasantness the world has offered up and we are trying to rationalise these hurts and misfortunes.

This naturally leads to the next step, which is plotting revenge. Some psychiatrists go as far as suggesting that perhaps our very favourite day dreams involve revenge fantasies.

Psychiatrists Mardi Horowitz and Susan Meffert have helpfully illuminated our grim desire for revenge in their chapter entitled 'Revenge Fantasies'[9] in the *Encyclopaedia of Stress*.

They argue that seething with anger has an energizing function, which can be therapeutic when we're feeling beaten up by the world, or our adversary. Nursing targeted anger encourages us to feel strong, while fear creates a sense of weakness and vulnerability.

Self-righteous indignation is popular across the media in general, and indeed many programmes, like talk radio shows – as Horowitz and Meffert point out – even seek to stoke it. These psychiatrists advocate caution in this regard, because revenge fantasies are easy to plant, yet hard to uproot.

Sometimes it seems as if whole professions (such as journalism, law and politics) are founded on exploiting our weakness for revenge.

Horowitz and Meffert suggest that after a betrayal, bitterness and resentment lead to self-righteous indignation, which then becomes difficult to shake off, because it feels so much like energy, or fuel for the soul. Burning anger makes us feel hard and solid, instead of puny, hollow or apathetic.

Is there a way out of this?

Breaking free of the revenge trap is possible, they argue, but psychological treatment, in their view, starts with the insight that we can be strong *without* self-righteous rage. Next we need to analyse our predicament, rather than replaying an endless loop of the revenge tape in our heads, which in reality goes nowhere.

After experiencing a traumatic betrayal, Horowitz and Meffert suggest asking yourself whether the perpetrator is an enemy or, perhaps, an unreliable narcissist.

Horowitz and Meffert believe escape from the revenge trap is only possible by avoiding demonizing the target of moral indignation (but is this what the press are up to today?). They are not suggesting passive resignation to enduring wrongs. Turning the other cheek, they acknowledge, may only invite more slaps in the face.

Giving up self-righteousness, they believe, is not the same thing as giving up moral indignation. Ethical outrage is a healthy response to seeing people break rules when they could follow them. Moral indignation is a motivating force in the world for good, but is easy to confuse with the desire for revenge. Someone who has been sexually assaulted, for instance, may deploy moral indignation, campaigning to counteract the exposure of others to abuse or neglect. This kind of exasperation, in the view of Horowitz and Meffert, is effective and adaptive, whereas chronic bitterness and revenge fantasies are ultimately unproductive.

One of the best ways, in our experience, to help those ensnared by the desire for retaliation is to explain that unless they forgive others (rather than seek revenge) their adversaries will continue to have power over them.

Horowitz and Meffert conclude that the most powerful antidote to revenge fantasy is a new adage: *When you feel bitter, do good.* Put another way: when you feel bitter, seek the good. They contend this is a variant to popular suggestions such as to perform random acts of kindness or senseless acts of beauty.

The psychiatrists' reasoning is that usually we want to be virtuous when we feel wonderful, as when we are in love. Their treatment for revenge rumination is to do good, particularly when we are more despondent. They contend bringing goodness into the world when we feel humiliated, affronted, fuming and unsatisfied most effectively counteracts self-righteous rage and revenge impulses.

'When you feel bitter, do good' works because it counteracts two customary but malignant reactions to being insulted. One response is to cave in and feel feeble, punctured, and degraded; the other is the opposite, a result of role reversal, to adopt a tough, menacing role, lashing out at others who are weaker.

The next time you are betrayed and start ruminating and plotting revenge, remember the advice from two world specialists on the subject – *when you feel bitter, do good.*

Is there really another way? Is it possible that ultimately the idea of trying to win the debate, to frame the argument as them and us, maintains a social distance which ultimately renders everyone a loser? That winning arguments or fighting with others is about trying to resolve hidden hurts? This may be particularly pertinent when we are facing such a serious threat as a pandemic.

Perhaps the most extreme example to make the point is what happens when the dispute you have with your adversary is so strong that reconciliation appears impossible. Should you, for example, forgive a mass killer who murdered your own son?

Mass killer Brenton Tarrant has just become the first person in New Zealand to receive a term of life imprisonment without parole. Given the heinous nature of the crime, the sentence was not a surprise. During the massacre on 15 March 2019 at two mosques, he fired at the injured, those hiding, running away, or calling for help; he even shot a three-year-old child. New Zealand does not have a death penalty.

But it was the heartfelt declaration of forgiveness, in court, by one bereaved mother, addressing the perpetrator of New Zealand's worst peacetime massacre, which has generated worldwide attention. During a series of victim statements, Janna Ezat, whose son Hussein Al-Umari was one of fifty-one people killed in 2019's Christchurch shooting, said to the twenty-nine-year-old 'white supremacist' about her son; 'He used to give me flowers for my birthday but instead I got his body...'

Then she looked up from the speech she had been reading, and gazing directly at the mass killer, declared, in what appears to have been an unscripted statement, 'I have decided to forgive you, Mr Tarrant, because I don't have hate, I don't have revenge, in our Muslim faith we say if we are able to forgive, forgive. I forgive you. Damage was done and Hussein will never be here so I have only one choice, to forgive you.' Tarrant, it is reported, appeared to nod, acknowledging her words, blinking profusely, then wiping his eyes.

But is this act of forgiveness letting the offender get away with their crimes?

The Hollywood film industry uses revenge as a leading plot device, suggesting these recurrent stories fill a deep need in our psyche. Psychologists find that plotting retaliation towards those who have wronged us occupies a surprisingly large part of our mental space. Maybe revenge fantasies are a good thing; perhaps they bestow a sense of restored purpose and control in an otherwise wrecked life.

Casey Ryan Kelly[10] has even recently mounted an argument that part of the psychology of President Donald Trump's appeal to his electorate centres on a widespread popular desire for vengeance, which his speeches, according to this theory, manipulate and exploit.

His analysis, entitled 'Donald J. Trump and the rhetoric of ressentiment', argues that Trump offers his audience an emotional-moral framework in which feelings such as anger, rage, malice and desire for revenge are never at rest, and no one act of vengeance can dissipate the nation's desire for more.

However, the pursuit of payback might also be dangerous for your mental health, trapping you forever in negative emotions flowing from a wound that you keep picking at as you contemplate retaliation. Maybe you can't get on with your life while you remain obsessed with getting even. To forgive has therefore traditionally been viewed by mental health experts as superior psychologically in the longer term, compared to obsessively plotting retribution.

It may have been a mistake to see forgiveness and revenge as opposing strategies; instead both might be empowering. The decisive issue is which strategy better restores a sense of power over your life. Being made to feel a victim is inherently damaging because it means control over your life has been taken from you. Power is liberating because it restores a sense of control.

Psychologists Peter Strelan, Jan-Willem Van Prooijen and Mario Gollwitzer[11] found revenge is empowering when the person who hurt you did so with strong intent to cause you harm. However, the authors also point out that revenge is likely to be unsatisfying when it serves no clear purpose. If victims can see that their wrongdoer understands the reasons for revenge, or has learnt from it, then revenge will help you feel empowered, resulting in better well-being. The study also points out that forgiveness can be empowering because experiencing wrongdoing is like being burdened with emotional baggage. When people forgive, they cast aside that weight; they are signalling that the terrible consequences of another's actions will not enslave them.

The new insight appears to be that revenge and forgiveness may both play a role in recovery. Pursue whatever strategy returns a sense of power and control over your life. Seeking revenge, if that desire merely ends up controlling you and producing no closure, in the end returns you back to victim status.

This study reveals the hidden psychological depths of the moment when Janna Ezat so poignantly said to Brenton Tarrant that she had no choice but to forgive. Her belief, and that of her faith, through which she had received the strength to survive, is that to embrace hatred instead might be a psychological trap from which there is no escape.

This statement of forgiveness appeared to wield particular psychological power, in particular appearing to move the killer when nothing else of the harrowing victims' experiences had throughout the trial.

One explanation is very surprising: that mass killers themselves are obsessed and controlled by revenge.

One motivation behind a particular sub-type – the so-called 'pseudo-commando' – is in fact being driven by a revenge fantasy that has become all-consuming.

James Knoll, a clinical professor of psychiatry and behavioural sciences, has described[12] how the pseudo-commando's pattern is to kill in public, to plan offences well in advance, with no escape planned, expecting to be killed during the incident. The pseudo-commando is driven by burning feelings of anger and resentment arising from feeling persecuted; he is therefore enacting a highly personal agenda of payback.

Perhaps Brenton Tarrant's apparent emotional reaction to Janna Ezat's statement was due to the idea that her faith had helped her survive mentally so that she might forgive. She was indicating the true strength of such a religious conviction, a power which mere psychotherapy can often only dream of, and which, therefore, could never be destroyed by mere physical annihilation, as he had attempted.

But maybe he was not sad for her, but instead was selfishly sorry for himself. His attempts to destroy this Muslim's woman's life, through taking her son, had in the end proved futile because she preferred to forgive.

Mass killer Brenton Tarrant got life without parole. Janna Ezat has chosen not to be imprisoned for life by hatred.

13

INSIDE THE MINDS OF THOSE TROLLING CAPTAIN SIR TOM MOORE

Does the pandemic and 'Tall Poppy' syndrome explain worsening online trolling?

Captain Sir Thomas Moore (30 April 1920–2 February 2021), popularly known in the UK as 'Captain Tom', was a British Army officer who raised, on one estimate, £39 million for charity approaching his 100th birthday during the COVID-19 pandemic. On 6 April 2020, at the age of ninety-nine, Moore began a charity walk, using a walking frame to assist, aiming for 100 lengths of his garden. His initial goal was raising £1,000 by his 100th birthday in aid of NHS Charities. But as the story of his efforts – herculean given his frailty and advanced age – gained attention across the world, 1.5 million individual donations poured in. Among many accolades and honours for his efforts, on 17 July 2020, he was personally knighted by the Queen at Windsor Castle.

He died on 2 February after battling COVID-19 and pneumonia. The extensive media coverage suggests he came to represent hope and resistance in the darkness.

Captain Sir Tom Moore's daughter has revealed in a TV interview with the BBC that the Second World War veteran was venomously criticised online for taking a holiday in Barbados over Christmas.

Hannah Ingram-Moore said that as the online trolling would have 'broken his heart', the family kept it from her father.

The Guardian reports that a hearing will take place on Wednesday at Lanark sheriff court in Scotland after a thirty-five-year-old man was charged in connection with an alleged offensive message posted on Twitter.

The ensuing Twitter storm over the story include suggestions that it was irresponsible of Tom Moore to travel to Barbados. Some have argued that Captain Tom's trip was in reality a public relations stunt with a hidden agenda by British Airways, promoting air travel during a pandemic.

But investigations into the psychology of trolling have found these posts are deliberately hostile with the precise aim to cause distress, or even psychological harm to the victims. Focusing on the particular content misses the psychological point of what is really going on.

Some 28 per cent of those surveyed in the USA admitted to malicious actions targeting strangers on the internet. Sadism was the best predictor of trolling, even more than narcissism, psychopathy or Machiavellianism, suggesting trolls basically derive pleasure and amusement from inflicting pain on others.

Trolling appears to be evolving from being 'for the Lolz', for laughs, to 'for the Lulz', which means more the joy of upsetting another's emotional equilibrium.

Within the gaming community, a new type of trolling is referred to as 'griefing'. Griefers aim purely to disrupt others' game experience, rendering the playing experience painful or even traumatic. This has become a form of entertainment.

Another new type of trolling, referred to as rest-in-peace (RIP) trolling, or memorial page trolling, targets those grieving online over the recent loss of a loved one by posting offensive and harassing comments designed to incite angry responses.

In the case of teenager Natasha MacBryde, her memorial page was trolled with disturbing images after she committed suicide. Similarly, in 2013, a memorial page created for Matthew Kocher on Facebook was inundated with posts mocking him after he drowned in Lake Michigan.

Both trolls and sadists feel glee at the distress of others.

Kathryn Seigfried-Spellar, a cyberdeviance expert, and Siddharth Chowdhury have recently conducted the first scientific investigation[1] into RIP trolling.

They found that 20 per cent of self-reported trolls have engaged in RIP trolling. Compared to 'mainstream' trolling, RIP trolls tend to score much lower on conscientiousness. They argued that the cluster of personality attributes they found meant that RIP trolls experience more feelings of dissatisfaction towards life compared to non-RIP trolls.

The authors of the study, entitled 'Death and Lulz: Understanding the personality characteristics of RIP trolls', argue that posting obscene comments on the memorial pages of deceased loved ones may be an emotional outlet for RIP trolls.

Those grieving for a lost loved one are signalling they indeed once had something precious to lose. Maybe they become targets because RIP trolls have never experienced an equivalent viable close relationship, or a functional, successful part of their life, so witnessing grieving ignites a resentment within them, which results in an aggressive retaliation?

Is there something unique to the UK about the phenomenon of Captain Tom Moore trolling?

A tendency to take pleasure in the failure of high achievers has been called *Schadenfreude*, a German word describing joy from witnessing another's failure.

The authors of 'Appreciation of achievement and a behavioural preference to view failure: *Schadenfreude* online'[2] argue that individualistic cultures (e.g. the USA) are more likely to favour the reward of high achievers.

The study used a psychological test referred to as the 'Tall Poppy Scale'. This assessed a preference for high achievers to succeed or to fail. Tall Poppy Syndrome refers to the expectation that poppies should grow together, so if one grows too tall it should be cut down to size. Previous research has found that those with lower self-esteem demonstrate a greater preference for high achievers to fail.

This new study, published in the journal *Personality and Individual Differences*, found that those with lower decisional self-esteem favoured the fall of the Tall Poppy. Decisional self-esteem refers to how effective people feel their decision-making is. Poor decision-making involves dysfunctional approaches such as procrastination and buck-passing.

Those who favour the fall of Tall Poppies are particularly interested in websites providing details of failures of others, and appear to like gloating at others' misfortune, particularly that of the successful.

The pandemic forced us all to make new decisions we never countenanced before. It tested our decision-making capacities. Adapting to unprecedented and challenging conditions usually meant relying on previous habits or choices to function, but in the pandemic this could not work. Not having to go to work daily, for example, in a lockdown, meant you were forced to make your own decision about when to get out of bed in the morning.

Poor decision-makers will have been particularly challenged and exposed by the pandemic. If impoverished decision-making produces a tendency to want to gloat over the previously successful enduring some kind of failure, then one coping mechanism the pandemic will have stoked is a new epidemic of internet trolling.

In order to maintain group cohesion, there may even be a preference for high achievers to fail in some cultures.

Captain Tom achieved something extraordinary, using nothing more than a walking frame and a back garden, because he made an amazing decision. That determination liberated him from all the restrictions imposed on him by a pandemic, his age and his vulnerability. By just walking back and forth, he stepped out of that garden and into Windsor Castle – and the world.

Some are going to find that resolution very threatening, and will retaliate. But this is just their way of dealing with their own demons.

The problem is they remain blind to what they could learn from Captain Tom, whose legacy could liberate them from themselves.

14

COPING WITH QUARANTINE

*The latest psychological research unearths some surprising
mental effects of quarantine*

One way of trying to achieve quarantine is to pelt your family with stones
if they approach you. They don't believe that you have coronavirus and
are trying to reason with you, yet you have become convinced you're
COVID-19 positive, and are desperate to keep them away to save their lives.

This is what happened to K. Bala Krishna in the Chittoor district of
Andhra Pradesh, India, in early February 2020.[1] The farmer was told by
local doctors on 5 February that he had contracted a non-specific viral
illness after developing symptoms of a cold and fever. He had not been
in contact with anyone who had coronavirus, and no such cases had yet
been reported in Andhra Pradesh or the adjoining area. At this stage, his
family reasoned with him that despite his fears, it was extremely unlikely
he had COVID-19.

This was right back at the beginning of the pandemic, when the main
information available appeared to be alarming videos of symptomatic
cases on the internet. Mr Krishna became obsessed with watching these.
They appeared to inflict a profoundly negative psychological effect on
him. The father of three became so alarmed at the prospect of infecting
his family that he sneaked out of the house on 10 February and bolted the
door from the outside, preventing his family chasing after him.

He was later found hanged from a tree near his mother's grave.

One of the most underestimated aspects of the virus, in terms of stress,
is the notion of quarantine. In the 2003 SARS outbreak in Taiwan, one of

the people trapped in a hospital during enforced quarantine also hanged themselves in despair.

Years after you have been released from quarantine, you can still suffer from profound psychological effects. Elevated rates of mental health problems, such as post-traumatic stress, depression and alcoholism, can all be traced back to the stress of confinement three years earlier.

These are the conclusions of a group of mental health experts[2] based in the UK (including a psychiatrist who had also served in the army, and who had been deployed to various hostile environments including Afghanistan and Iraq). Their study was published in one of the oldest and most prestigious medical journals in the world, *The Lancet*, and attempted comprehensively to review the body of previously published scientific research into psychological survival of quarantine.

This investigation found profound impacts on lives, beyond the issue of mental health, after the quarantine was over. For example, weeks after being released from quarantine, avoidance behaviour in healthcare workers persisted, such as minimising direct contact with patients and not reporting to work.

Other research cited by this study found 54 per cent of people who had been quarantined avoided those who were coughing or sneezing, 26 per cent avoided crowded or enclosed places, and 21 per cent avoided all public spaces in the weeks following the quarantine period. For some, the return to normality was delayed for many months.

This investigation reviewed evidence that governments should be cautious about introducing quarantine given that some of the effects can be counter-productive. For example, one study argued that travel bans and other lockdown measures may inadvertently spread disease, because the economic hardship induces an unintentional consequence of increasing the migration of potentially infected people from affected areas.

One of the studies examined the enforced quarantine of a hospital in Taiwan following a SARS outbreak there in 2003.[3] All 930 staff were ordered into a two-week quarantine, yet were expected to perform duties as usual. All 240 patients staying at the hospital were banned from leaving, as were 129 visitors and outpatients.

Everyone was imprisoned in the hospital for at least fourteen days while the police cordoned off the building. After watching some healthcare workers die from SARS, some medical staff tried to escape, while others refused to provide care for the ill. Telephone lines and television cables were cut by the authorities – citing security reasons – adding sheer terror to the mental duress of the lockdown. One nurse tried to leap out an eighth-floor window before being restrained by colleagues.

The authors of this investigation into the Taipei Municipal Hoping Hospital SARS quarantine of 2003[4] point out that the full psychological impact was revealed when on just the third day of confinement a depressed man who was suspected of having SARS hanged himself. This was despite psychiatric counselling. The following day, another suicide attempt was halted when a patient was prevented from jumping out of a window.

The Lancet study quoted an investigation[5] into the stress of quarantine following a 2007 outbreak of highly infectious equine influenza in Australia, which found that those with one child had a 20 per cent higher risk of significant psychological distress than those with no children. Yet this study, entitled 'Factors influencing psychological distress during a disease epidemic: Data from Australia's first outbreak of equine influenza', also found that having three or more children appeared protective against severe psychological distress.

Perhaps having more children represents a distraction from the monotony of quarantine, though it's hard to get one's head around the idea that more children in this circumstance would not be a nightmare. One joke which did the rounds on the internet early in the pandemic was that if the doctors didn't develop a vaccine soon, the parents would step in and do it for them.

Another possible explanation for this intriguing finding is that having three children simply might mean being older. The study found one of the primary factors associated with severe psychological distress during an epidemic was age. Those in the 16–24 age category reported the highest levels of psychological distress.

It could therefore be that post-quarantine it is the young who appear to need the most psychological support. We might lose a whole generation, psychologically rather than virally, to this pandemic. The elderly may be most vulnerable to physical attack from COVID-19 but it is the young who might be least immune to the longer-term mental effects once quarantine is over.

Another possible explanation for this fascinating finding is suggested by some other research[6] where the precise opposite occurred to the usual quarantine procedure being reported here: people were quarantined because attempts were being made to infect them deliberately.

'Parenthood and Host Resistance to the Common Cold' investigated immune resistance to viruses by quarantining subjects, then administering nasal drops containing one of four common cold viruses. They were then monitored for the development of a clinical cold.

The intriguing finding is that the more children you have as a parent, the more resistant you are to getting the common cold. One possible explanation is that you have built up immunity over time because you have more children, and children constantly expose you to bugs.

Another reason this might be an important link with psychological resilience during quarantine is that *The Lancet* review[2] found a major cause of psychological strain was becoming worried if physical symptoms potentially related to the infection were experienced. This fear that the symptoms could reflect having the infection continued to be related to mental health difficulties several months later. It might be that parents with lots of children, having been through the mill with infections being brought home, are better set up for quarantine because they are already more resigned or resilient or immune, and therefore either shrug off ambiguous or irrelevant symptoms, or just don't get them.

We all get physical symptoms quite a lot of the time, but usually these just go away of their own accord, and so we give them little attention. During quarantine, in contrast, we become hyper-vigilant for signs we have got the thing we were being quarantined against, and this constant worrying about what the latest symptoms mean might take a more significant toll on our mental health than previously appreciated.

As the physical symptoms of anxiety can look very similar to a viral infection – for example, headache, difficulty breathing, or hyperventilation and a cough – it is possible to enter a panic cycle. Your anxiety makes you believe you have the viral infection you dread as you detect physical symptoms attributable to rising panic but mistake them for the flu. You get more panicky and descend into a spiral of ever-increasing mental and physical distress.

This cycle is worth remembering in our current pandemic.

K. Bala Krishna,[1] the farmer from India who hanged himself after becoming preoccupied with internet videos about COVID-19, may have found himself caught in this panic cycle. Perhaps if this had been explained to him at the time he might be alive now.

The conclusion of the just-published academic investigation[2] in *The Lancet* argues that 'altruism is better than compulsion'. The authors contend that superior coping with the mental strain of such confinement could also hinge on whether or not those quarantined are motivated to comply because of a sense of volunteering, and free choice, seeing meaning in their sacrifice by assisting others. If we are being *compelled* to endure the many different sacrifices of quarantine, without it being clear exactly why it's necessary, then poorer coping and worse mental health becomes more a more likely outcome.

It may be important for our resilience to try to retain a sense of both purpose and perspective on our fears.[7]

PART 2

SHOULD YOU ALWAYS DO
WHAT YOU ARE TOLD?

15

DOES LOCKDOWN INFLICT THE SAME MENTAL HEALTH EFFECTS AS IMPRISONMENT?

Why do some ex-cons reveal that lockdown is more challenging, in many ways, than incarceration ever was?

Is the impact of the lockdown on our mental health being underestimated or, even worse, systematically ignored by our government? Could our leaders be motivated for political reasons to underplay the psychological damage of their policies?

A new study[1] comparing the psychological impact of lockdown on the general population in the UK and California with the mental experience of prisoners banged up in medium-security prisons finds that people in lockdown reported feeling more hopeless than first-time prisoners. This is particularly worrying as feelings of hopelessness are directly linked to suicidal thoughts and another recent study has forecast 100,000 additional suicides worldwide because of the pandemic.

As the UK is already at the top or near the top of the league table for deaths related to COVID-19 per head of population, might we be on course for a similarly tragic league-topping result when the suicide and mental illness statistics are finally collated? Should we wait for that, or should we now be debating whether lockdown policies adequately take into account the mental health impact?

Academics at Middlesex University, London, and Leeds University Business School conducted their prison comparison study because the experience of enforced confinement of the general population has led some to liken lockdown to imprisonment. The authors directly compared the general public's suffering during lockdown with prisoners' experiences of imprisonment. The research investigated whether psychological parallels could be drawn between these two forms of confinement.

The researchers acknowledge that although governments introducing lockdown policies do not intend to punish their citizens as courts do when sending convicted offenders to prison, such policies can have tragic inadvertent consequences. Can psychological parallels be drawn between the two forms of confinement?

The research found that people in lockdown in both California and the UK were also significantly less engaged in a range of daily activities than were first-time prisoners. Is the government commissioning enough research and investigation into exactly what is happening inside people's homes during lockdown? This study found that although males in lockdown had, on average, more interaction with those in their living space than did first-time prisoners, both groups had a similar frequency of contact with family/friends from the outside.

'Are People Experiencing the "Pains of Imprisonment" During the COVID-19 Lockdown?' involved a survey of 300 adults in lockdown in the UK and 450 adults in lockdown in California. Data were collected in the UK and in California in April 2020. This was approximately four and five weeks after the first lockdown began in each region, respectively. The survey results were compared to 267 prisoners from two medium-security prisons in England, and 307 prisoners from a medium-security federal prison in California.

The prison data were collected before the current pandemic, so the prisoner's experience is not influenced by any current COVID-19 outbreak in the prison system, nor by the prisoners being psychologically influenced by lockdown in the outside world.

The study found that females in lockdown in both the UK and California thought about being attacked/beaten up as often as did first-time prisoners. The authors point out that prisons are notoriously violent places, so the COVID-19 lockdown may have had a dramatic effect on violence that occurs within the home.

The research also uncovered that the sorts of activities believed to enrich prisoners' lives and help them cope with their confinement (e.g. education and self-help programs) were less prevalent in the public during lockdown.

Most concerning was the finding that people in lockdown felt more hopeless relative to before lockdown compared to first-time prisoners before they went to prison. The authors argue their results are compatible with the growing body of research reporting severe mental distress suffered by those enduring lockdown.

As such feelings of hopelessness are predictive of suicidal thinking, attempted suicide and death by suicide, others have similarly forecast increased suicides worldwide.

Following the great recession of 2008, there was a dramatic increase in suicides in North America and Europe: an extra 10,000 people in those regions killed themselves between 2008 and 2010.[2]

These shocking results came from a study published in the *British Journal of Psychiatry* which demonstrated that using statistical and comparison techniques it was possible to confirm that the economic downturn had contributed to a raised suicide rate. The study, entitled 'Economic Suicides in the Great Recession in Europe and North America', also figured out how many of the additional suicides were linked to the recession.[2]

But the current pandemic is predicted to produce a global economic meltdown of much greater breadth and depth than the recession of 2008. So how many more people might kill themselves as a direct result?

Professor Carl Weems, Bethany McCurdy and Mikaela Scozzafava from Iowa State University, and Professor Victor Carrion from Stanford University, have conducted a study which suggests that, depending on levels of unemployment and its duration and the duration of isolation, even 100,000 extra suicides worldwide is possible.[3] However, the authors are also keen to emphasise that their numbers are just a forecast, and that they should be used with a view to acting now to prevent the statistics ever reaching that scale. Their current forecast is for the raised suicide rate to endure for up to two years from now.

In some ways, prisoners are actually psychologically better off than the public experiencing a lockdown. Prisoners at least know when their sentence will end, and also have to obey a set of rules which, while horribly restrictive, tend not to change dramatically, let alone reverse every few weeks.

One of the comments posted under a version of this chapter I published on a medical website included the reaction of an ex-prisoner who had been 'inside' for around fifteen years. He had in fact enjoyed training and education opportunities in prison. He was even befriended and supported by an Anglican chaplain. After release, he engaged further with the faith community. He explained that lockdown had been more challenging, in many ways, than incarceration ever was.

Another comment pointed out that hotel quarantine has the potential to be even more damaging than incarceration, as it can include two weeks of solitary confinement. UN rules on the treatment of prisoners forbid solitary confinement with no outside time for exercise. The individual points out that they would have been better off if they had punched the policeman in the airport and got sent to jail rather than hotel quarantine!

16

PSYCHOLOGISTS PREDICT PUBLIC REBELLION WILL ERUPT AGAINST THE LOCKDOWN

Will it, if the government continues to follow an out-of-date psychology strategy?

The next time you stay at a hotel, be careful about the review you leave on a site like TripAdvisor. Believe it or not, the wrong kind of review could land you in jail.

Perhaps hotels are more frazzled in a post-lockdown world and nervous about negative reviews given how difficult it has been to keep afloat in the pandemic. That is one possible explanation for what happened to Wesley Barnes, who visited Sea View Resort in Thailand in June 2020.[1] He did not appear, from his subsequent negative reviews on TripAdvisor, to have enjoyed himself.

His one-star review of the property was headlined 'Unfriendly staff and horrible restaurant manager'. Below that he posted:

Unfriendly staff, no one ever smiles. They act like they don't want anyone there. The restaurant manager was the worst. He is from the Czech Republic. He is extremely rude and impolite to guests. Find another place. There are plenty with nicer staff that are happy you are staying with them.

The hotel then alleges that Barnes wrote another now-deleted review, which carried an allegation of 'modern slavery'. It turns out Thailand has very strict anti-defamation laws, and the resort reported Wesley to the police for defamation. They claim he refused to take down the alleged inflammatory review after repeated requests and warnings.

He was arrested in September and then spent two nights in jail, while facing two years in prison for the allegation. TripAdvisor paid his legal fees and he was released, though the dispute continues, as can be seen from the current posting TripAdvisor placed over the resort's listing on their site:

> This hotel or individuals associated with this hotel filed criminal charges against a TripAdvisor user in relation to the traveller writing and posting online reviews. The reviewer spent time in jail as a result. TripAdvisor serves its users best when travellers are free to share their opinions and experiences on our platform – both positive and negative. The hotel may have been exercising its legal rights under local law, however, it is our role to inform you so you may take this into consideration when researching your travel plans.

This true story is a good example of what happens if you use coercion to get people to comply. Sometimes, this strategy backfires spectacularly. However, I for one always leave five star reviews now at any resort I attend, just to make sure I can get to the airport without being detained.

Perhaps governments on a pandemic planet have all begun to behave a bit like some resorts in Thailand?

A psychological turning point in this pandemic always appears to be just around the corner: the point when lockdowns become ineffective because of widespread public rebellion. How many more sacrifices can the public make? Even a relatively minor rebellion has the potential to put the whole country at risk, psychologically fracturing community solidarity, perhaps irrevocably.

We were told as the first lockdown in the UK started that because the Prime Minister, through illness, was indisposed, the decision to review the lockdown was to be postponed. This apparently innocuous statement reveals much about the behind-the-scenes psychological reasoning over how to maintain national acquiescence.

At first glance, this comes straight out of spin manipulation lesson number one: use a delaying tactic to avoid doing something you never wanted to do anyway (lift the lockdown), buying you time, attributing it to circumstances which are difficult to quibble with – i.e. the need for the Prime Minister to recover.

Part of this strategy placed a lot of store on the authority of Boris Johnson to secure obedience from the public. The outpouring of goodwill towards the sick premier was perhaps deployed for political ends. However, the current reliance on 'obedience' and 'authority', which seems to be driving these tactics behind closed doors in Whitehall, is in fact based on a largely discredited theory of behavioural science.

This flawed approach strains the relationship between the ruled and the ruling class, possibly to breaking point. Astute handling of the emotional aspect of this problem remains imperative to securing continuing compliance from the nation.

The results of the most famous experiment in the history of the behavioural sciences, Yale psychologist Stanley Milgram's 'shocking', notorious 'Obedience to Authority' experiments,[2] suggest that popular obedience could decline dramatically, particularly if the government continues to follow its current emotional course. The lessons of these experiments, conducted in the 1960s, about securing co-operation and how easily it can be lost, hold the key to saving quarantine now.

In Milgram's study, members of the public were persuaded by white-coated authority figures to administer seemingly life-threatening electric shocks to strangers. But the subjects remained unaware that the person receiving the shocks was in fact part of the experiment, merely play-acting the effects of electrocution.

And yet 65 per cent of the public went all the way up to administering such a high voltage that the experimenter's 'subject' appeared to have been rendered unconscious, or possibly dead.

The astounding power of the authority figure to secure blind obedience seemed to be confirmed. For the first time, credence was now lent to the previously incomprehensible claims, during the Nuremberg Trials, of so many 'ordinary Germans' that they were passively following Nazi orders to murder innocents.

The authority of the white-coated academic and scientist is particularly apposite right now.

It is no accident, if you have read the Milgram experiments, that our ministers are always flanked by professors and doctors. Our government invokes the authority of the white coat to secure blind obedience, exactly as Milgram's experiment indicated.

But this strategy misunderstands the real lesson of the most influential, yet notorious, obedience experiment of all time.

The future of quarantine restrictions and popular revolt is going to turn on the issue of whether we are being encouraged to engage with our leaders in a joint enterprise, a shared vision, or whether we are, as their messages get more strident and demanding, in effect being ordered to obey.

This interpretation of the experiments was recently published at the University of Queensland, Australia and the University of St Andrews in Scotland.

Psychologists Alexander Haslam and Stephen Reicher's conclusion[3] is that almost completely the opposite and wrong lesson may have been traditionally drawn over the population's inclination blindly to obey authority figures.

In their new investigation, published in the academic journal *Annual Review of Law and Social Science*, they argue that when one looks closely at what actually happened during the experiment, as opposed to what most *think* happened, it was not in fact ordering the public that achieved cooperation.

Polite requests were how the experimenter began dealing with non-compliance (just as our government began asking us to remain home), becoming increasingly forceful before culminating in a direct order.

Is this the same journey that our leaders are on?

This new investigation, entitled, '50 Years of "Obedience to Authority": From Blind Conformity to Engaged Followership', found that it was the direct order, of all the different persuasive verbal 'prods', which was in fact *most likely to be disobeyed* by subjects in the Milgram experiment, almost the opposite of the message conventionally taken away.

It was instead a subtle yet more powerful psychology: the identification of the subject with the joint enterprise, in Milgram's case, to apparently further the cause of the scientific discovery. The subjects bought into the idea that they were sharing a joint mission with the experimenter, and that was why they 'obeyed'.

The compelling evidence is that giving people a direct order is one of the least effective ways of securing their compliance. There is no natural, widespread tendency to instinctively obey commands from authorities. Instead, participants in the 'obedience to authority' research are most biddable when encouraged to continue *for the sake of the experiment*. They are most likely to comply when they are invited to cooperate in a joint enterprise *which they believe in*.

Haslam and Reicher have conducted separate experiments which suggest that those who don't, for example, subscribe as much to the scientific outlook, nor the scientific enterprise, may not be as liable to identify with the project of the white-coated expert, and are not, therefore, as likely to be obedient to people in white coats.

This highlights another deep psychological problem with the government's persuasion strategy: it appears founded upon the conviction that the public will continue to obey the scientists and mathematicians, because somehow the average person identifies with a scientific project based on official statistics. This appears to be a woeful misunderstanding of the average person's relationship with science and maths as a guide to life.

It is therefore possible we are being led by people in power who are being influenced by an out-of-date and wrong-headed psychological basis for the strategy of getting the nation to comply.[4]

Even more worrying is Haslam and Reicher's conclusion that ordering people to do things can backfire and generate more non-compliance.

A clue that this thesis may be coming true might be found in the evidence that the government's repetitive injunctions seem to be less effective over time. As the mandarins blindly worship at the altar of 'obedience to authority', the danger is that this might provoke a yet more authoritarian response.

The Economist reports[5] that Google's smartphone data confirms that Europe's second lockdown in the autumn of 2020 had much less impact on daily life compared to the first in spring.

There certainly seems to be an erosion in the enthusiasm for following restrictive rules. If public perception is growing that no one in government is enduring the same consequences which they are expecting the ordinary public to suffer, this will create a mental obstacle to convincing us we should all continue to subscribe to 'sharing' lockdown.

How long can the myth that this is a genuine 'joint project' continue to be sold to a public being ordered to take shock after shock as the government ramps up the voltage?

17

CAN DOMINIC CUMMINGS' MINDSET EXPLAIN LOCKDOWN LAXITY?

If you can't see that senior Downing Street advisers breaking lockdown rules will eventually produce a public rebellion, then you need your eyes tested

Under the headline[1] 'Top officials around the world keep getting caught breaking lockdown rules', *The Washington Post* listed several examples from the early days of the virus, including Austrian President Alexander Van der Bellen apologising for violating his government's own rules by staying out significantly longer than was allowed. Another apology was issued after Polish Prime Minister Mateusz Morawiecki sat too close to several non-family members in a restaurant while no one wore a mask.

The Washington Post cited the example of UK epidemiologist Neil Ferguson, an important senior adviser to the British government on its coronavirus response, who resigned after it was revealed that he broke lockdown edicts when a woman described as his lover visited him at home. It was Ferguson's own research which drove official policy to adopt strict isolation measures.

Can psychology explain this pattern of the otherwise politically astute and successful breaking rules so clumsily and obviously, then facing the career-ending glare of media and public scrutiny?

Is it simply the case that the pandemic has inadvertently revealed something many already suspected: that political elites believe there is one rule for them, and another for the rest of the population? Appearances of solidarity are deceptive, and basically no matter what the propaganda slogans say, we are not 'all in it together'.

One of the most salient examples of this syndrome was that of Dominic Cummings, former special adviser to UK Prime Minister Boris Johnson, who attempted to defend his apparent breaking of lockdown rules. In late March, he drove 260 miles from London to Durham with his ill wife and their young son, in apparent direct contravention of the government's urgent message to stay home, especially if coronavirus symptoms are present.

The grave danger with the special adviser defending his having broken lockdown rules in late March and early April is that it plays directly to the question of whether the UK, as well as the rest of the world, is being governed by political elites who are never committed to the rules they issue while expecting the lower orders to follow them.

Conservative MP David Warburton,[2] as reported in *The Guardian*, described how his father had died alone as a result of following the rules and declared Cummings's actions gave the impression of 'double standards'. He told the BBC:

> People have made sacrifices, this is a difficult time … in those sacrifices there really hasn't been the choice to use instinct. Instinct hasn't really been part of it. We've been tasked with following regulations laid down by the government.

This goes to the heart of the issue from a psychological standpoint: is it the case that the political elite in the UK, and maybe elsewhere, rely on instincts when it comes to ethical behaviour (Dominic Cummings explained that he didn't feel the need to consult with the Prime Minister, possibly suggesting he thought that his instincts would be shared by his boss), which is at variance with those of the public?

Because instincts by definition operate at such a basic psychological level, our ruling elite may not even be fully aware of the way in which they differ from the rest of us.

Dominic Cummings did seem bewildered during and after his unprecedented press conference by the strength of reaction to his attempted defence. This is all the more surprising for someone credited with masterminding the latest electoral success of the government.

Dr Nicholas Allen and Professor Sarah Birch have published academic research[3] which has found that candidates for parliamentary office in the UK display significantly more tolerance of ethically dubious behaviour than members of the public. Within the elite category, elected MPs exhibit more permissive ethical standards than those candidates who are unsuccessful.

The study, entitled 'On either side of a moat? Elite and mass attitudes towards right and wrong', included a reference to a previous political scandal where members of the UK parliament appeared to be abusing their parliamentary expenses allocation by, for example, claiming for the purchase of a duck island and the cost of cleaning a moat.

The study found that sitting MPs and Conservatives (both in and out of the UK House of Commons) appear to be significantly more tolerant, compared to the public, of ethically questionable behaviour. This had also been found in previous research conducted in the late 1980s. The authors conclude: 'There is something about the ideology of the modern Conservative Party – or some other shared characteristic of Tory politicians – that makes its MPs and prospective MPs more tolerant of ethical deviance than other political belief systems.'

The study points out that one way of thinking about corruption is that it falls into 'black', 'white' and 'grey' categories. 'Black' corruption refers to behaviour that both the public and political elites agree is clearly improper. 'White' corruption, in contrast, refers to acts generally tolerated by both groups.

Crucially, between 'black' and 'white' lies 'grey' corruption, which elicits different reactions from elites and citizens. Perhaps this is the territory in which Dominic Cummings' lockdown behaviour resides.

Political scientists contend that a majority of one group (the public) might regard behaviour lying in the 'grey' area as being extremely corrupt, while a majority of the other (e.g. political elites) might genuinely regard it as being only marginally reprehensible, or else be ambivalent about its significance.

Nicholas Allen and Sarah Birch's research involved putting several possibly morally questionable political acts to the 2005 British Representation Study (BRS), a survey of all major-party candidates, including incumbent MPs, conducted at the time of the 2005 general election, as well as to a representative survey of the British adult population conducted by YouGov in April 2009.

Whilst there was agreement between political elites and the public in several areas on what counted as unacceptable corruption, significant gaps opened up between the groups on some scenarios. These included a chair of a company being given an honour in return for that company making a big donation to a political party; a minister using influence to benefit a firm in his or her constituency; and a Member of Parliament being retained to arrange meetings and dinners in the House of Commons. In response to these particular scenarios, the large majority of the public declared this behaviour corrupt, while much smaller proportions of candidates and MPs said the same.

They nevertheless point out that it is not the case that political elites could be generally described as morally bankrupt. Indeed, in some situations political elites take certain rules even more seriously than the public, often when dealing with unambiguously illegal acts.

Also, political elites are aware of the fact that there will be interference in their personal lives and sacrifices as a result of entering politics. For example, previous research has found that political elites and the public agreed about what was ethical in such scenarios as a cabinet minister not telling the prime minister about seeing a psychiatrist.

This research has nevertheless confirmed that the moral instincts of political elites and the public do part ways in certain significant predicaments. It does appear that those are the quandaries that arise when political elites are more aware than the general public of 'how politics works' on the inside; in other words, how political advantage is obtained behind the scenes in the real world.

Political scientists refer to 'volitional' failures, when individuals consciously decide to act improperly, in contrast to more 'cognitive' failures, when individuals believe themselves exempt from moral requirements.

It could be that the Dominic Cummings incident is more an example of a 'cognitive' failure in that, according to this research conducted by Nicholas Allen and Sarah Birch, his world outlook is shaped by his background in politics, leading him to a different understanding of what to do when the situation is ambiguous, at least in his eyes. They conclude that their results support the theory that politicians as a class are more tolerant of ethically dubious behaviour when there is ambiguity. It might be that the journey to power warps ethical standards.

The theory that political elites suffer 'cognitive' failures is hugely significant to the predicament of Dominic Cummings and to the government. When our leaders are deciding to impose severe lockdown rules on a country, causing widespread public suffering, do they do so believing the same rules will apply to them? If our political elite believed harsh restrictions also applied to them equally, and were more aware of the severe personal implications and consequences, might they actually have come up with a different policy?

It might however be the case that it wasn't so much Dominic Cummings' specific actions as it was his poorly constructed and bizarre excuse which actually landed him in much more trouble. Cummings defended his breaking of lockdown rules with the excuse that he drove to Barnard Castle to test his eyesight as he had to drive back to London later.

As previously mentioned, Neil Ferguson, an eminent academic who was pivotal to the government's lockdown policy, also appeared to be yet another highly intelligent authority figure who displayed a lamentably poor grasp of how to make a valid excuse.

He was revealed to be receiving visits from a lover in the midst of lockdown. The professor said at the time of his resignation, 'I acted in the belief that I was immune, having tested positive for coronavirus and completely isolated myself for almost two weeks after developing symptoms.'

Yet it was his modelling that had led to a national lockdown, during which his actions of connecting with another person were specifically prohibited, regardless of testing positive or not. It appeared to betray to many sections in the press an imperious, *de haut en bas* approach by our political elites. (See chapter 18 for more on Neil Ferguson's actions.)

Back in 2013, the Mayor of Toronto, Rob Ford, who died in March 2016, reportedly explained his taking of crack cocaine as down to being in a 'drunken stupor'. Following the release of a video portraying an agitated Mr Ford vowing to rip out someone's throat, poke out their eyes and ensure they were dead, it was reported he was considering 'rehab'. Protestors in Toronto who wanted him to resign held up signs to TV cameras explaining, 'I'm not at work today because I'm in one of my drunken stupors.'

Excusing alleged crack cocaine abuse by being in a drunken stupor may appear, at first glance, a poor strategy, yet psychological research confirms that well-made excuses generally work. But excuses are only therapeutic if they help us skate over a temporary glitch. If we rely on excuses to constantly wriggle out of trouble, then pretexts become dangerous.

At the heart of the pandemic has been a new problem: it has provided a host of new excuses for poor performance by those who were always looking for an escape from their jobs or responsibilities. Everyone who ever wanted to avoid work or targets now has COVID-19 to blame. The epidemic has led to the rise of a new excuse culture.

Psychologists Barry Schlenker, Beth Pontari and Andrew Christopher published one of the most comprehensive academic reviews[4] of what makes a 'successful' excuse, but cautioned that in our society the cry of 'it's not my fault' was becoming an all-too-common refrain even before this new pandemic arrived.

The then Mayor of Toronto may not have realised that psychologists have uncovered that there is an art to constructing excuses that reliably get you out of trouble. Many now appear to be working harder at excuses than their actual jobs, but how to give a really good excuse still eludes most.

The authors of the paper point out that an effective defence is designed to convince audiences that, to the extent that you *are* at fault, the blunders derive from less 'central' aspects of character (i.e. from carelessness rather than stupidity).

Their review, entitled 'Excuses and Character: Personal and Social Implications of Excuses', points out that a poorly made excuse leaves the culprit appearing deceitful, ineffectual and self-absorbed to the detriment of others. Bad excuses dig you further into the hole you were trying to wriggle out of.

Professor Barry Schlenker has pioneered a simple technique called the 'The Triangle Model of Responsibility', which provides the scaffold on which effective excuses are constructed. Schlenker contends that responsibility is the basic psychological glue that connects us to a bungle.

The three components of the Responsibility Triangle are (a) prescription clarity – how clear were the rules that applied? Examples of excuses in this category are underperforming students' explanations that 'the objectives of the class were unclear so I didn't know how to get a good grade' or 'the instructor never explained what would be covered on the test'.

The next arm of the responsibility triangle is (b) personal obligation, the extent to which you were bound by the rules. Examples of such excuses, according to Schlenker, Pontari and Christopher, are, 'That wasn't my job, it was his,' 'I'm too young to be considered responsible for murder,' 'I don't have to follow those rules because I'm the boss's son,' and 'I couldn't complete the assigned task on time because my first duty was to resolve a family emergency.'

The final arm of the responsibility triangle is (c) personal control. For example, failures can be attributed to external circumstances that wrested control from you ('The dog ate my homework'). Internal states can similarly have deprived you of control ('I do poorly on that type of test because of my learning disability,' 'I couldn't help it, I was drunk') or a combination of both ('I cheated on my spouse because I was psychologically abused as a child and developed an uncontrollable desire to be loved').

Schlenker, Pontari and Christopher point out that all superior pretexts will make effective use of at least one arm of the Responsibility Triangle.

The authors contend that for excuses to work they first must be credible. Secondly, excuses must maintain self-engagement in cases of important recurring tasks. The excuse of being in a drunken stupor, given a mayor has to continue doing responsible work, won't really cut it for an electorate. Thirdly, excuses must maintain goodwill for the excuse-maker, and not give the impression of self-absorption.

Effective excuses work because they permit the excuse-maker to maintain the appearance of having integrity and being effectual and concerned with the greater good (upholding important principles, caring about others), rather than being cripplingly self-absorbed.

Having illuminated how to make effective excuses, the authors question whether there hasn't been a general growing societal tendency to shift blame and not take responsibility. We appear to have become a culture where a litany of excuses is deployed to explain away transgressions and failures. The proclamation 'It's not my fault' is everywhere. They argue that if we don't take responsibility for our lives and therefore our errors, we become unreliable.

Being reliable means that others can depend on us. Being reliable often involves personal costs, such as keeping one's word even when it might be more profitable in the short run to break it; expending extra effort, even when quitting is easier; or acting to take into account others instead of focusing solely on one's own welfare.

The grave danger of excuses is that they carry the serious potential to undermine reliability. Once reliability is undermined, then society ceases to function.[5]

The late Rob Ford was quoted by the BBC as explaining back in 2013, 'I am only human,' which might be the ultimate fall-back excuse. He reportedly added: 'Yes, one day I do want to run for prime minister.'

18

THE PSYCHOLOGY
BEHIND NEIL FERGUSON'S
RESIGNATION SCANDAL

*The press puzzle over why Professor Neil Ferguson broke UK
lockdown rules*

Professor Neil Ferguson, whose statistical modelling prompted the UK
to go into lockdown, resigned from his government advisory positions
after *The Daily Telegraph*[1] revealed that he had been flouting official
isolation rules in order to meet his married lover. The fifty-one-year-old
epidemiologist apparently allowed the thirty-eight-year-old woman to
visit him at his home during lockdown while he publicly preached
the need for strict social distancing during the pandemic. *The Daily
Telegraph* reported that the woman apparently crossed London to visit
the professor at least twice during lockdown, which is against the very
regulations the professor's own research had brought about.

The policy was inspired by his estimate that half a million UK citizens
might die from the pandemic without lockdown measures. This dramatic
number came from the computer-modelling team which he led at
Imperial College London. *The Daily Telegraph* reported that the former
government adviser was married with a son, but that he and his wife lived
apart; however, the press also appeared puzzled that such an eminent
mathematician could have so foolishly destroyed his national reputation,
which had accrued over many years. Exactly why did he violate the very
rules he seemed so passionate about, endangering the credibility of his
own advice – and, most importantly, threatening public confidence in the
lockdown?

Journalist Paul Nuki writing in *The Daily Telegraph*[2] speculated that Neil Ferguson was 'felled by a risk-taking character streak and overactive libido'.

Evolutionary psychology predicts that some men pursue high office precisely in order to gain access to the kind of desirable women they wouldn't otherwise attract.[3]

Many evolutionary psychologists argue somewhat controversially that we are driven by forces beneath our conscious awareness, suppressed by the veneer of civilization. Evolution, so the argument goes, has shaped our DNA over many generations, meaning we choose mates most likely to disseminate our genes. Who we fall in love with is not up to our own individual aesthetic preference, but instead reflects a chromosomal choice.

One aspect of these theories is that men have inherited a biologically based proclivity for sex with as many different women as possible; whereas women are genetically programmed by a contrasting sexual selection strategy: namely, investing in fewer relationships, but with longer-term commitments, as this aids the survival of their offspring.[3]

Women, in contrast to men, are looking for a higher quality but lower number of different relationships. This kind of theorising, which is essentially predicated upon gender differences, is controversial among psychologists and is regarded in some quarters as the height of political incorrectness.

According to evolutionary psychology theory, men are drawn to youthful appearance because of the concomitant advantages to fertility. On the other hand, women value character traits, like ambition and intelligence, which lead to status and wealth. For a woman, the theory goes, this brings material advantages for her children; but her attraction to these characteristics in men operates below conscious awareness. Women are not aware of the reasons why they find these features in men desirable; just as men are equally victims of, or slaves to, the biology which shapes their sexual behaviour and preferences.[3]

A university professor who has become a national figure and who advises the government becomes attractive to women, according to evolutionary psychology theory, because of his intelligence and status (and indeed, perhaps wealth will follow).

One evolutionary psychology study,[3] entitled 'Teaching may be hazardous to your marriage', found that college professors are at greater risk of being divorced or separated. This 'politically incorrect' study argued that these older men are exposed to younger women on a daily basis in the form of students. The younger women are genetically programmed to be attracted to high-status males – for example, senior eminent academics – rather than their younger, lower-status, male counterparts.

The study argued that college professors' more mature wives appear less physically attractive to the senior academics, and as a result professors' commitment to their marriage subsequently wanes. For the same reason, the study argued, in comparison with other divorced men, divorced college professors appear less likely to remarry.

This study was inspired by previous research which found that men who were exposed to photographs of physically attractive women subsequently became less satisfied with their current heterosexual relationships, and rated their partners less attractive.

The college professor study contends that the daily exposure to young women draws a male college professor's attention to the contrast between the physical appearance of younger women – which men's evolved psychological mechanisms find more attractive – and that of older women like their spouses. This sharp contrast, according to the study, then produces discontent in the man's mind, and it is this dissatisfaction, rather than the younger women themselves or affairs with them, that simultaneously leads to an increased risk of divorce or separation and a decreased probability of remarriage.

The college professor study analysed one of the largest social science data sets, the General Social Survey, collected from 1972 to 1996, constituting 532,845 subjects representative of non-institutionalized adults in the United States.

The results are that simultaneously being male and a college professor significantly increases the statistical likelihood of being divorced.

However, a later study,[4] entitled 'One woman's behaviour affects the attractiveness of others', suggests that the differences between genders on this question of attractiveness may be more fluid than evolutionary psychology predicts.

The researchers asked participants to view upper-body photographs of highly attractive opposite-sex underwear models, obtained from men's and women's underwear catalogues. Unattached participants then viewed opposite-sex 'average-looking' photographs. They were then asked whether the pictures of the average-looking people met the participant's threshold for a potential date. Women, more than men, showed a sharper drop-off in desire for the average-looking men after seeing highly attractive pictures of the opposite sex.

In other words, when women are exposed to physically attractive men, they then find the average man less desirable; and this shift in 'contrast effect' desire was stronger for women than for men in this particular study.

However, this study went on to examine the impact of being exposed not to physical attractiveness but instead to a receptive member of the opposite sex who is 'moderately attractive'.

Pairs of videos were shot featuring the same actor in each. But they differed in that in one the actor behaved receptively towards the viewer: smiling, looking directly at the camera, and generally acting as if encouraging future interaction. In the comparison video, the actor behaved unreceptively: never smiling, gaze wandering, and sounding bored.

When exposed to these two different videos, men were more likely subsequently to differentially down-rate their current partners (or other opposite-sex people) more than were women, on the basis of attractiveness.

That is to say, mated men's ratings of their partners, and unattached men's ratings of other women, were both *lower*, if the interviewee had smiled and acted warmly, than if she seemed uninterested. Women exhibited no such effects after watching a male interviewee.

The authors argued this might be because it is more adaptive for men to detect and respond to receptive behaviours, as this leads to a more successful allocation of their mating effort. To the male brain, such signals may indicate an immediate potential mating opportunity. Their results suggest that males, more than females, shift their preferences in order to allocate mating effort toward immediate courtship targets.

Evolutionary psychology predicts this sex difference, because indicators of interest from the opposite sex are rarer, and therefore of more value for men than for women.

It is argued that high-status men like those in Neil Ferguson's position historically repeatedly risk (and eventually lose) prestigious government jobs in order to conduct relationships of this sort; and so this is not, to them, a puzzle at all.

They contend that men worked very hard to achieve high status 'precisely so that they could gain intimacy with a woman who looks like this one', as one evolutionary psychologist actually said to me. They therefore contend that it would have been a greater puzzle if a man in a position like Neil Ferguson's *hadn't* had relations with such a woman merely because he had attained an important government position and part of his job was to tell everyone to stay home.

The downside of evolutionary psychology is that it can appear to provide excuses for behaviour that may have had its explanation in terms of the 'law of the jungle' but is not helpful now that we have become more civilised, and have higher aspirations to transcend our 'animal' programming.

The virus is genetically programmed to attack us; our only defence appears so far not to be our own biology, which in fact seems vulnerable to this threat. Instead, we must unleash our best brains to attack it with superior medicine and technology.

But we won't defeat the disease if we allow another part of our biology, our emotional drives and weaknesses, to determine who is on our front line. There is natural indignation and *anger* at an authority figure breaking the law. Psychology can help us see how common inner conflicts that are part of human nature can lead to rule-breaking and political self-destruction. Psychology can help us *forgive*, thus keeping the allies we really need on our team.

For us to lose possible valuable scientific insight just because we are unforgiving of fallibility, which could be part of all of our genetic and psychological make-up, may also be our own undoing.

In that case, it wouldn't be the virus that killed us, but our own inner psychological enemies.[5]

19

DID COVID KARMA KILL TRUMP'S CAMPAIGN?

Are presidential elections decided by candidates' apparent health?

Is it possible that Donald Trump's COVID-19 infection was the significant turning point of the US Presidential election, because of its psychological impact on voters? Is the virus determining who gets elected and therefore who runs our lives?

The answer to this question may lie in what happened to Hillary Clinton, Donald Trump's rival in the last presidential election, back in 2016, where she suffered a health scare with remarkable parallels to current events.

In the last few weeks of the 2016 presidential campaign, Democratic Party nominee Hillary Clinton departed early from a memorial service. Footage posted on Twitter showed her surrounded by Secret Service agents as she left, requiring assistance as she stumbled to a van.

The video went viral and forced her personal physician to report that the candidate was diagnosed with pneumonia, and had become dehydrated. The incident became a pivotal turning point in the campaign – according to an Economist/YouGov poll, in just under a week the percentage of Americans who felt Clinton was in 'good enough physical condition to effectively serve as president' dropped from 52 per cent to 39 per cent.

Maybe it was the pneumonia which killed her campaign?

A CNN Poll conducted by SSRS in the days following the announcement that the President had contracted COVID-19 found that two-thirds of Americans say President Donald Trump handled the risk of spreading coronavirus infection to others around him irresponsibly.[1]

Ryan Neville-Shepard and Jaclyn Nolan have recently published an in-depth psychological and sociological analysis[2] of the Hillary Clinton sickness scare. They argue that public perception of candidates' health can have dramatic repercussions, including determining the outcome of an election. Such scares can have a great impact on voters' perceptions of who has the stamina for the job of president.

Entitled '"She Doesn't Have the Stamina"': Hillary Clinton and the Hysteria Diagnosis in the 2016 Presidential Election', the study points to other precedents, like the infamous Thomas Eagleton incident in the election of 1972. Senator Thomas Eagleton, the running mate of Democratic nominee George McGovern, was found to be suffering from bipolar disorder. Reports of Eagleton's condition caused the McGovern campaign to panic, forcing Eagleton's resignation.

The authors of this latest analysis ask why Clinton's 'overheating incident' marked such a turning point in the presidential campaign, when the USA went on to elect a man they contend was clinically overweight, averse to exercise, suffering from high cholesterol, and devoted to fast food.

Perhaps Donald Trump was more alive to the profound psychology behind how health is communicated, or demonstrated to the public – hence his reassuring drive-past in a motorcade to wave to his supporters when not yet discharged from hospital during the 2020 campaign. Perhaps in terms of voter psychology, it didn't matter that this may have been a medically dangerous act towards the other people in the car.

But maybe Trump was sealing his fate more than he realises in merely wanting to be re-elected?

Neville-Shepard and Nolan quote from a study[3] entitled 'The mortal presidency: Illness and anguish in the White House', which found that, excluding four assassinated presidents, all of the remaining holders of the office 'together paint a striking picture of premature death'. Despite higher life expectancy for people in their social class, and top-notch medical care once they become president, almost two-thirds have died prematurely.

One theory about why this is focuses on the stress of the job.

The art of handling the stress requires the ability to repeatedly turn reversal of fortune into an asset, something Hillary Clinton perhaps never quite mastered. Maybe it's no accident that Donald Trump had deftly attempted to turn falling ill into a strength, referring to how he had 'learned a lot about Covid' and that this was the 'real school'. He also strode out of the White House to the helicopter taking him to the hospital as opposed to being videoed covertly stumbling as did Hillary Clinton.

In a phone-in interview with Fox Business Channel during the 2020 campaign, President Trump said: 'I'm back because I'm a perfect physical specimen.'

Back in the 2016 presidential campaign, Donald Trump's former physician promised Trump would be the healthiest president ever, yet later confessed that his hyperbolic letter had been dictated by Trump himself. Speaking with CNN's Anderson Cooper, Clinton complained that 'Trump's doctor said he'd be the healthiest president in history. That's just not even serious.'

Yet maybe in the war of words and public perception over candidate's health Hillary Clinton never really grasped psychologically what Trump had understood – how to deftly exploit the emotion behind presidential health.

For example, appearing on Fox News shortly after Clinton's emergency exit, Trump stated, 'I hope she gets well soon.' He then quickly added, 'Something is going on but I just hope she gets well and gets back on the trail.' Appearing magnanimous and generous also involved hinting that she might be very ill.

Neville-Shepard and Nolan point out in their analysis that the conspiracy theorists rapidly took over; video of Clinton leaving her daughter's apartment was interpreted as revealing that the campaign was using a body double. The healthy Hillary who emerged had a different nose, her earlobes had somehow changed shape, her index finger was a different length, and she had apparently lost weight.

Neville-Shepard and Nolan quote a study[4] entitled 'The health of the president and presidential candidates: The public's right to know', which concluded that: 'The things we want to know about the health of Presidents and presidential candidates tell us much more about ourselves than about the Presidents and would-be Presidents. They tell us what we fear.'

They argue that the real reason Hillary Clinton's campaign was undone by a health scare was in fact because many Americans still fear strong women leaders, and public obsession about their health says much more about contemporary gender bias than it does about a candidate's actual stamina to lead.

Another theory about our preoccupation with illness in our leaders is that it is not so much about physical fitness, but more about 'looking fit' – that is, 'fit' as per the modern slang, which is more a reference to sexual or physical desirability.

A recent study[5] found that politicians on the right of the political spectrum, on average, look more 'beautiful', a finding replicated in Europe, the US and Australia. The authors argue that as beautiful people typically earn more, they are more likely to oppose redistribution and so tend to end up on the right of the political spectrum.

The study contends that in an election where the voters don't know much about the political differences between individual candidates, then the superior physical attractiveness of those on the political right will result in an electoral advantage. The study also found that better-looking politicians are inferred by voters to stand further to the right, independently of which party they really represent.

Another recently published study,[6] 'Why are right-wing voters attracted to dominant leaders? Assessing competing theories of psychological mechanisms', argues that voting preference has a lot to do with the emotional way you view the world. Using state-of-the-art face-morphing software called Psycho Morph, the conductors of the study morphed pictures of Norwegian male politicians to look more or less facially dominant to investigate the impact on voting preference.

The authors argue that because politically right-wing people view life as fundamentally more hazardous, beset with conflict between rival groups, this explains the conservative preference for more dominant candidates. It appears more likely to lead to the survival of the followers given a dangerous world where, in the minds of such voters, dominance equates naturally to competence. The authors cite previous psychological research which finds that Republicans are perceived as more powerful than Democrats, who, in contrast, appear warmer.

The authors argue that the right-wing preference for dominance arises from the notion that, in a world full of enemies, the essential quality such voters are looking for in a leader is the aggressive overpowering of adversaries. This theory suggests election results might hinge on whether the virus was psychologically seen as an enemy to be overcome.

The results of their research suggest that while leaders of conservative parties might need to send indicators of dominance to attract their natural followers, such signals will in fact hurt leaders within liberal or left-wing parties because of the contrasting world view of their electoral base.

In 'Election systems, the "beauty premium" in politics, and the beauty of dissent',[7] researchers found that in German parliamentary elections the more physically attractive members of parliament, once elected, tended to dissent more often from the party line. This finding is one of the rare examples of research that helps voters figure out how a candidate is going to perform once elected.

Maybe the political impact of a political leader catching COVID-19 also has something to do with the way their doctors react. But, despite appearances to the contrary, physicians also suffer from fears too. VIPs in the public eye might in the end suffer worse treatment than the ordinary patient.

Doctors could be frightened of the reputational implications following the death of a famous patient, or too keen to chase the accolades for getting a celebrated personality back on their feet. Such excessive fears or ambitions generate over-treatment, which then becomes more hazardous than the underlying illness.

During the 2020 campaign, after being admitted to hospital with COVID-19, Donald Trump appears to have received a surprisingly extensive and intensive set of medical treatments for somebody who was supposedly not that unwell. His medical team declared that he had no symptoms, but the media have questioned whether he might still have been contagious.

Maybe in the end it is the narcissism of their doctors which draws leaders into trouble when they fall ill.

When Boris Johnson needed to be hospitalised, the doctors and nurses looking after him found themselves suddenly in the national media spotlight, just as Trump's doctors did. The intense and complex relationship between an ill patient and their physician thrusts the leader of a country into what can become an uncomfortable psychological predicament.

Mental health experts who have studied the national psychological impact of a political leader falling ill predict that much hinges on their personality and leadership style.

This is especially true in the midst of a national catastrophe, like the one we face now in the UK. A leader falling ill at an inopportune time can profoundly alter how the crisis is handled.

Two experts who have analysed in depth over forty cases of chiefs of state stricken by illness are Dr Jerrold Post, Emeritus Professor of Psychiatry, Political Psychology and International Affairs at George Washington University (who also worked for the CIA, psychologically analysing foreign leaders), and Dr Robert Robins, Professor Emeritus of Political Science at Tulane University.

These experts published studies[8] in the academic journal *Political Psychology* and elsewhere, and a book entitled *When Illness Strikes the Leader*,[9] in which they argued that sometimes a leader's illness can by itself alter the course of history.

The dynamic that develops between an inner circle and a weakened authority is essential. For instance, a leader who already tended to delegate to their inner circle may engender a protective attitude when they fall ill. But if the leader's narcissism meant they retained power jealously, not listening to advice, then their illness can become disastrous for their country.

Post and Robins argue that a disease with a fluctuating course might become particularly troublesome for the leadership's inner circle, and therefore potentially most hazardous for the nation. This is especially so when the person in charge is in denial over the true extent of their disability.

Partially disabled leaders might be more manipulated when in a weakened state; those pursuing power in the inner circle will then seize the opportunity provided by a temporary incapacity. But Post and Robins also warn that subordinates who act too assertively when the leader is weakened may find themselves out of favour (and a job) when the leader improves. A reshuffle in senior roles shortly after a leader recovers betrays what really happened around the leader's hospital bed.

Post and Robins describe an especially dangerous psychological syndrome which they have seen develop repeatedly which they term 'The Captive King and His Captive Court'.

This is a particularly unhealthy dynamic in which disastrous decisions are more likely to be made as the leader and the inner circle do not really trust each other, yet each needs the other to survive politically.

The deep psychological implications of a leader falling ill can reverberate unexpectedly. For example, the medical care leaders receive historically has been distorted by their fame and power. This is reflected in the name of this section of Post and Jerrold's work: 'Being a VIP May Be Hazardous to Your Health'.

While our media kept reporting the party line that Prime Minister Boris Johnson was receiving excellent care in order to reassure the nation at this psychologically threatening time, clinicians are only human and can also be affected by this kind of particularly high-stakes illness. According to Post and Robins' investigations of this clinical predicament, doctors treating a national leader under such pressure can disagree more than usual about the diagnosis and correct course of treatment.

Boris Johnson's particular personal hero, Winston Churchill, of whom he was so enamoured that he even wrote a biography, *The Churchill Factor: How One Man Made History*, may have suffered from exactly this phenomenon of significantly altered medical treatment.

According to a study entitled 'Did Winston Churchill suffer a myocardial infarction in the White House at Christmas 1941?',[10] Dr Allister Vale and Dr John Scadding explored a medical incident that might have changed the course of the war. While staying in the White House over Christmas 1941, Churchill apparently developed chest pain. Sir Charles Wilson, his personal physician, diagnosed a heart attack. But Wilson, possibly for political and personal reasons, decided not to apprise Churchill of this diagnosis, nor even to obtain support from US medical colleagues. Instead, Dr Wilson waited until Churchill's return to London before seeking a second opinion.

If Dr Wilson had been dealing with any other patient, and if this patient had not been the Prime Minister in the midst of a war that was not going well, might the physician have immediately admitted Churchill for precautionary investigations, fundamentally altering the course of history? Do doctors of leaders take into account the political implications of treatment and diagnosis, so altering their normal hospitalization plan?

Psychologists who conduct experiments investigating how our preferences for leadership qualities change when our society is facing external threat – war, for instance – find that at those times we retain a deep psychological tendency to look for more dominance and strength in a leader.[11] We even prefer leaders who just *look* more physically formidable when we find ourselves facing an external threat.[11] Evolutionary psychologists have argued this is an almost genetic drive evolving to promote survivability because of our violent ancestral past.

This psychological perspective suggests that when citizens most need to respect and obey the authority of government, for example over complying with quarantine restrictions, sickness and therefore weakness in a commander might be disastrous.[12]

Even if a leader makes a successful recovery from an ailment, if it was serious enough to remind them of their mortality, this in itself can have a profound psychological impact, changing them personally, possibly forever.[13] Jerrold Post and Robert Robins argue that following an illness, narcissistic leaders consumed by dreams of glory may become particularly driven by a sense of mission.

A sense of urgency to accomplish goals before 'time runs out' means that, after an illness, a personal timetable might start to take precedence over a nation's longer-term interests.

20

DOES THE PANDEMIC MEAN THAT THE FUTURE IS NOW FEMALE?

Why do female leaders appear to have been more effective?

Finland has a coalition government led by five women. Thirty-four-year-old Sanna Marin became the world's youngest serving prime minister in 2019. Her government attracted admiration for its early response to COVID-19. This female leadership locked down the country in mid-March 2020 with just under 300 recorded cases of the virus at that time.[1]

During the first half of 2020, two countries declared the pandemic effectively over: New Zealand and Iceland. At that time both had either no new cases of COVID-19 infection or too few to consider the epidemic as continuing.

At the time of writing, Taiwan had reported nine deaths and an even lower COVID-19 incidence rate (20.7 cases per million) compared with NZ (278 per million).[2]

All these countries are led by women. Is this a coincidence?

The Daily Telegraph in the UK declared at the beginning of the pandemic that four of the top ten countries with the lowest death rates and best virus testing have women in the highest job: Taiwan, New Zealand, Iceland and Estonia. Also commended on their country's superior pandemic performance was Angela Merkel's Germany, and Denmark, led by Mette Frederiksen.[3] The title of the article was 'Why do female leaders seem so good at tackling the coronavirus pandemic?'

Meanwhile in the UK, Boris Johnson was presiding over the highest predicted death toll across Europe. According to Johns Hopkins University at that time, the UK already had the world's highest observed case-fatality ratio, the number of deaths per 100 confirmed cases.

Boris Johnson at this time also celebrated the birth of his sixth child, the product of apparently his third long-term relationship, following two previous divorces. Maybe he reflects the stereotype of 'old school' masculinity. His oldest child, Lara, at twenty-seven years old, is just four years younger than Ms Symonds, his fiancée.

Another unapologetically old-style male is Donald Trump, running the White House and presiding over the highest number of deaths in any one nation worldwide. Yet his country expends more on health than any other; spending per person in the USA is 28 per cent higher than Switzerland, the next highest per capita spender. Trump has five children from three marriages.

Is the pandemic revealing the deficiencies of male leadership compared to the benefits of having a woman in charge? After the disease retreats, will the future become more female?

The virus already kills more men than women, but is it also butchering the cigar-chomping Churchillian idea that belligerent male leaders are tougher in a fight to the death?

Forbes magazine[4] entitled its take on this subject 'What Do Countries With The Best Coronavirus Responses Have In Common? Women Leaders', and declared:

> From Iceland to Taiwan and from Germany to New Zealand, women are stepping up to show the world how to manage... Add in Finland, Iceland and Denmark, and this pandemic is revealing that women have what it takes.

Both *The Daily Telegraph* and *Forbes* emphasised supposedly feminine qualities, such as greater empathy and a more caring, collaborative spirit, as explaining the female edge. *Forbes* invoked the example of Norway's Prime Minister, Erna Solberg, who held a televised press conference devoted just to children; no adults were allowed.

Yet the fundamental reason female leaders seem to be making better decisions than their male counterparts facing the same pandemic crisis appears to be because these women are being more decisive and tougher than male commanders.

New Zealand's Jacinda Ardern's famous mantra has been 'go hard and go early', imposing a strict lockdown four days before the first COVID-19 death in her country. Tsai Ing-wen in Taiwan introduced over a hundred measures to block the contagion in January, leading CNN to admire her country's response as one of the world's best.

Female national leaders did indeed lock down their countries earlier and suffered half as many COVID-19 deaths on average as male leaders, according to an academic analysis comparing nearly 200 countries.

Professor Uma Kambhampati, head of the School of Politics, Economics and International Relations at the University of Reading, conducted a study[1] with Professor Supriya Garikipati, an economist at the University of Liverpool. Professor Kambhampati commented: 'This study is the most comprehensive yet of the human decisions being made by global leaders to deal with the COVID-19 pandemic. Our analysis shows that the decisions taken to lockdown countries earlier by their female leaders has saved lives.'[5]

Professor Supriya Garikipati[5] argued:

> Our results clearly indicate that women leaders reacted more quickly and decisively in the face of potential fatalities. In almost all cases, they locked down earlier than male leaders in similar circumstances... While this may have longer-term economic implications, it has certainly helped these countries to save lives, as evidenced by the significantly lower number of deaths in these countries.

Only nineteen of 194 countries were led by women but on average these countries locked down after significantly fewer deaths than countries led by men. The women are better at being proper 'men' than their male counterparts, in terms of strength of character and boldness; this is the theory that comes from a group of psychologists who have been studying female leadership for over a decade.

The publication[6] is entitled 'Getting on top of the glass cliff', and refers to a 'glass cliff' that confronts women climbing the greasy pole in organisations. It greets them after they have smashed through the infamous 'glass ceiling', an invisible barrier of prejudice keeping them from opportunities for advancement.

This research began with a finding that prior to the appointment of men onto the board, FTSE 100 companies on the London Stock

Exchange typically experienced stable share prices, yet in sharp contrast, in the five months *prior* to the appointment of a woman, companies had endured poorer share price performance. Another study examined loss-making companies listed on the London Stock Exchange. This showed that if the loss was 'big', these companies subsequently had increased gender diversity on their boards compared to non-loss-makers. The implication is that men have fewer qualms appointing women into leadership roles when they think the position is something of a poisoned chalice.

The 'glass cliff' phenomenon can be found in politics as well. Archival analysis of the 2005 UK general election found that within the Conservative Party, female candidates contested seats that were significantly more difficult to win because the candidate they were up against had won a higher proportion of votes at the previous election.

It was through an even more hostile environment in the UK in the 1970s and 1980s that Margaret Thatcher battled to become one of the most electorally successful Conservative prime ministers ever. Yet she took over leadership of a party and country in crisis; the Conservatives had just unsuccessfully fought two general elections in one year, and their previous prime minister had introduced the three-day working week to cope with an unprecedented economic and political predicament.

One theory to explain this finding, according to these researchers[6], is that predicaments facilitate risk-taking, allowing organisations to try something new, or to question the status quo. Such emergency situations open up previously unavailable opportunities for women to take on leadership positions. Also, when a company is in crisis, appointing a less stereotypical leader becomes a signal to stakeholders that change is being introduced. And women may be more willing than men to accept leadership positions in times of crisis because they have relatively few opportunities to reach the top: beggars can't be choosers.

These researchers map the path to power for women as profoundly different to that of men. Women get their breaks because they are routinely handed a difficult predicament; to succeed they have to overcome higher hurdles than men. Perhaps this then renders them stronger psychologically.

For example, Jacinda Ardern took over the leadership of the New Zealand Labour Party in 2017 following the resignation of its former leader because of poor polling. She was invited to head an organisation in crisis, exactly as would be predicted by the 'glass cliff'. A mere two months afterwards, in a stunning turnaround, she was elected the country's youngest prime minister in 150 years, and its youngest female PM ever. Her meteoric rise coined a new term: Jacindamania.

The 'glass cliff' means that female leaders have literally been 'tested' more, ensuring cooler heads under pressure. It is not that female leaders are necessarily more empathic or collaborative, or caring, which is in fact old-fashioned gender stereotyping belonging to a pre-COVID-19 era. Instead it is their contrasting *experience* which generates their competitive edge.

A threat that hits everyone at the same time, like a pandemic, is a kind of unique, planet-wide political experiment, allowing us to compare our systems and societies in an unprecedented manner. What the virus has illuminated more than was ever possible before – because its rapid lethality has stripped away the previous immunity provided by spin and the careful use of PR – is how much leadership is really about character.

Boris Johnson and Donald Trump, in the style of some more typical male characters, have contagiously jumped from relationship to relationship, marriage to marriage. Their aura has meant they keep getting second and even third chances (a bit like the virus in their countries). Men at the top are not generally 'tested' in the same way as their female counterparts; instead, they are 'indulged'.

This contrast has now been exposed because COVID-19 remained stubbornly unimpressed and indifferent to macho posturing.

In the end, the virus test has revealed a 'pre-existing condition' we may otherwise have never noticed: that some male leaders enjoy a plumped-up cushion rather than facing a glass cliff.

A study[7] examining all the countries involved in international conflicts around the world over the last fifty years found that the more women were involved in the leadership of a society, the less militarily aggressive that society was, and the lower the probability of violent conflict with other countries.

The researchers argue that their study, in the *Journal of Conflict Resolution*, is strong evidence for the proposition that, generally, women work for peace and men wage war. Women are more likely to use a collective or consensual approach to problem-solving, rather than focusing on the unilateral imposition of solutions.

Psychologically, at quite a profound level, the authors suggest, men tend to engage in power struggles for personal gain, whereas women tend to attempt to minimise power differences, to share resources, and to treat others equally. Yet despite these advantages of female leadership, by the time the study had been completed in 2001, only twenty-four countries around the world had placed a female leader in office since 1900.

The study, entitled 'Gender, violence, and international crisis', found only 16.6 per cent of these countries led by a woman were involved in international crises at any point during the period of female leadership, and none of these female leaders initiated the crises.

The researchers used political equality, measured as the percentage of women in parliament, as a measure of gender equality within society. Put simply, their finding is that as the percentage of women in the legislature of a country increases, the less severe is the violence between countries. Indeed, if the percentage of women in the legislature increases by 5 per cent, a state is nearly five times less likely to use violence internationally. In terms of the current warlike position of the USA compared with more pacifist Europe, it is interesting to note that the USA had far fewer women in its legislature compared with most European countries – for the USA the figure was just over 14 per cent compared with Sweden at 42 per cent at the time this study was published.

Indeed, Scandinavian countries generally take the top six consecutive spots in the world league table for highest female representation in parliament – followed by Germany with 32 per cent in 2001. The UK, which has arguably been more aggressive in recent conflicts than the rest of Europe, was down at 17.9 per cent.

The authors, based at the University Minnesota and the University of Connecticut,[7] argue that competition, violence, intransigence and territoriality are all associated with a male approach to international relations. Women, on the other hand, are less likely to see crisis negotiation as a competition or to advocate the use of violence.

That said, Mary Caprioli and Mark Boyer argue in their study that female leaders are often perceived to be just as aggressive as men. Leaders of recent years such as Margaret Thatcher, Benazir Bhutto, Indira Ghandi and Golda Meir were seen as hawks rather than doves, and all were caught up in violent conflicts.

Perhaps female leaders must also contend with negative perceptions from male opponents. For example, gender was a factor in the events and resolution of the 1971 Indo-Pakistan war in which Indira Ghandi had an essential role. Caprioli and Boyer remind us that President Yahya Khan of Pakistan stated that he would have reacted less violently and been less rigid as the leader of Pakistan in the conflict with India if a male had headed the Indian government. Indeed, President Khan was quoted as saying: 'If that woman [Indira Gandhi] thinks she is going to cow me down, I refuse to take it.' The behaviour of male leaders when faced with a female opponent becomes a factor – a sense of macho pride which makes them unwilling to 'lose' to a woman, lest their masculinity be questioned.

Female leaders who have risen to power through a male-dominated political environment may well need to be more aggressive than their male counterparts in crisis according to Caprioli and Boyer. Although differences exist in male and female leadership styles, women in positions of power may find themselves compelled to convey their strength in traditional male terms. And they may also work harder to 'win' in a crisis for the same reasons, because to respond in a more feminine way would be seen as 'weakness' and would be political suicide.

Caprioli and Boyer's research suggests that we don't just need more women in parliaments and legislatures, but also to live in societies that embrace more feminine values, so that women who succeed will feel less pressure to be more like men.

This view is supported by Ruut Veenhoven,[8] a leading expert on happiness, who recently published a study with Willem Arrindell that found people in richer countries are happier in more feminine nations. The authors define masculine cultures as those which expect men to be assertive, ambitious and competitive, to strive for material success, and to respect whatever is big, strong and fast.

In these cultures women serve and care for the non-material side of life, for children and the weak. Feminine cultures, on the other hand, define relatively overlapping social roles for the sexes: men need not be ambitious or competitive but may go for a goal other than material success; men may respect that which is small, weak and slow.

One sign that you are living in a more feminine society by this analysis is if there is less occupational segregation; more male nurses, for example.

The study found that in more masculine cultures (such as Japan, Austria and Venezuela) political and organisational values emphasise material success and assertiveness, whereas in more feminine cultures (like Sweden, Norway and the Netherlands) they accentuate other values: interpersonal relationships, sympathy and concern for the weak.

If people are happier in feminine societies and if these countries tend to get involved in less conflict with their neighbours, maybe the enhancement that will produce the most well-being in the future would be for us to become in some senses more feminine.

This, in the sense conveyed by this research, means more empathic, kind and caring, more aware of others' emotional states and more able to influence our own and others' emotions.[9]

Another theory about the possible benefit of more feminine values in a country, argue Arrindell and Veenhoven, is that it may create greater opportunities for combining multiple social roles (employment, marriage, parenthood). The possibility of combining multiple roles is likely to make life more satisfying, in particular for women. The occupation of multiple social roles has been found to be associated with good physical and mental health in both women and men.

If the election of a female leader reflects a society embracing more feminine values, then this, according to the latest psychological research, appears to bode well for that country's future as regards waging war and general happiness.

The two candidates for the leadership of Britain in 2016 were the only two candidates left competing for the post in the Conservative Party leadership contest, and these were both women: Theresa May and Andrea Leadsom. However, they appeared to be descending into a typically masculine aggressive scrap. One salvo in their battle for power was the alleged accusation that one woman had children and the other didn't, and that this somehow mattered in how they were going to lead. Possibly a combative political system shapes our leaders more than their gender or any other factor.

Instead, most of all, we could ask a deeper question – by what *kind* of woman or man are we being led?[10]

PART 3

HOW FAR AWAY IS THE END?

21

WILL COVID STRESS HAVE AN IMPACT ON FUTURE GENERATIONS?

Could the pandemic have repercussions for decades to come?
Will children born now develop into adults shaped by the stress
they experienced in the womb?

Carrie Symonds, the fiancée of Boris Johnson, gave birth to a healthy baby boy despite carrying her pregnancy through a worldwide viral pandemic, her own social isolation and the father of her child being admitted to intensive care.

Boris Johnson has revealed to the UK press just how close he came to dying from the virus, even describing how contingency plans were drawn up for the eventuality of his death. Carrie Symonds would have had to contend with the fear of her fiancé's demise.

There is evidence that the sort of distress experienced by Carrie Symonds and by many other women during their pregnancies might lead to increases in mental health difficulties in children years later.

Petra Persson and Maya Rossin-Slater published an investigation[1] that seems to predict that the future mental health of children born to pregnancies during this pandemic may have been at least partly determined already. The study appears to predict a potentially significant spike in future mental health problems for the coronavirus generation.

The study was entitled 'Family Ruptures, Stress, and the Mental Health of the Next Generation', and found that if a mother suffered the stress of a bereavement during her pregnancy, in particular the death of a maternal relative, then the child she gave birth to was, years later, much more likely to be prescribed ADHD (attention deficit hyperactivity disorder) medications during childhood. Even into adult life, there was a significantly increased chance of being prescribed anti-anxiety and anti-depression medications.

At the time of writing, the 2.75 million mark has been reached in deaths worldwide linked to COVID-19, so, statistically speaking, many of these will have affected a pregnant woman close to the person who died.

While Carrie Symonds – and many other pregnant women – did not have to grieve for the death of the father of her child, when she experienced him fighting for his life she was put under the kind of strain which surely comes close to the levels of tension people experience during an actual bereavement,[2] and which many other pregnant women are enduring at this time, for various reasons.

The study,[1] published in 2018, investigated children born in Sweden between 1973 and 2011. Children whose mother lost a family member (a sibling, a parent, a maternal grandparent, the child's father, or an older child) in the nine months after the child's date of conception were investigated.

The investigation found that in utero exposure to the death of a mother's close relative during pregnancy has substantial effects on the children born. There were significant increases in later consumption of prescription drugs to treat mental health conditions both during childhood and even into adulthood.

For children, these effects include a 25 per cent rise in the likelihood of taking a drug used to treat ADHD, and a 24 per cent increase in the average daily dose of ADHD medications.

For adults, who had been in utero when their mothers experienced the bereavement, there was a 13 and 8 per cent increase in the likelihood of consuming prescription drugs for anxiety and depression respectively, as well as 19 and 12 per cent increases in the average daily doses of these medications. These effects are stronger when the deceased is a close relative of the mother.

These findings are especially relevant for the 'coronavirus generation' being born now and over the next few months, because the authors went on to calculate the impact of the strain of unemployment on pregnancy, and many millions of people all over the planet are going to find themselves unemployed or facing similar stresses as a result of the economic consequences of the pandemic.

Extrapolating from their findings and using data that come from other research, the authors calculate that in utero exposure to stress from unemployment leads to a 17.3 per cent increase in the likelihood of ever purchasing a drug to treat ADHD in middle childhood, and a 16.6 per cent increase in the average daily dose. There are also 9 and 5.5 per cent increases in the likelihood of ever purchasing drugs to treat anxiety and depression in adulthood respectively, and 13.1 and 8.3 per cent increases in the average daily doses of anti-anxiety and depression medications.

Other research has also established a link between mothers' cortisol (a stress hormone) levels during pregnancy and their children's future mental health,[3] suggesting there are plausible mechanisms that can account for these findings.[2] According to another separate study, pregnant women's exposure to the stress of the Six-Day Arab–Israeli War increased the likelihood of their children developing schizophrenia by the age of thirty.[4]

Another study investigated blood test evidence of prenatal influenza in mothers as the cause of schizophrenia in their children. Entitled 'Serologic evidence of prenatal influenza in the etiology of schizophrenia', the researchers based in the USA investigated those born from 1959 through 1966, and followed up for psychiatric disorders thirty to thirty-eight years later.[5] Archived maternal serum was assayed for influenza antibodies in pregnancies giving rise to offspring with schizophrenia. The risk of schizophrenia was increased seven-fold if the mother experienced influenza exposure during the first trimester of a pregnancy.[5]

Craig Garthwaite, an economist from the University of Maryland, has published a study investigating the so-called 'fetal origins hypothesis' in relation to the Spanish Flu epidemic.[6] The theory is that malnutrition or other complications, such as may occur because of a pregnant mother catching a viral illness or something similar, causes the foetus to shift blood and nutrients from vital organs to the brain.

This diversion is an attempt to protect the growing baby and improve the chances for survival, but leaves certain organs pre-programmed for failure in later life, often after fifty years or more.[6] This analysis of

384,000 observations found in utero exposure to the 1918 flu pandemic had long-lasting negative health consequences. Depending on the period of foetal development during which exposure occurred, individuals born to mothers pregnant at the time of the Spanish Flu epidemic had a higher probability of developing coronary heart disease, diabetes, kidney disorders, or being in poor health decades after the pandemic was over.

Another study, 'Does in utero exposure to illness matter? The 1918 influenza epidemic in Taiwan as a natural experiment', found those who were in their mother's womb during the pandemic ended up shorter as children/adolescents, and less educated.[7] They were also more likely to have serious health problems including kidney disease, circulatory and respiratory problems, and diabetes in old age. Even if the mother and child survive, there is a strong negative impact of in utero exposure to influenza.[7]

Surely Carrie Symonds experienced the compensatory euphoria of discovering her partner survived and didn't die, unlike the tension faced by the bereaved mothers in Persson and Rossin-Slater's research, so perhaps the mother of the Prime Minister's son faced less stress overall? But it is the issue of emotional turmoil which appears to be the big factor in disturbing a pregnancy. This means that enormously positive events, if they cause intense moods, also appear to have an effect.

A study[8] from the University of Colorado has examined the effect of US Super Bowl exposure on low birth weight, finding that first-trimester exposure (first three months) to the Super Bowl is associated with a 2 per cent increase in the probability of low birth weight (defined as weighing less than 2,500 grams at birth). Remarkably enough, first-trimester exposure to a Super Bowl win is associated with an almost 4 per cent increase in this probability. These percentages may appear small but they are statistically significant, and multiplied over thousands of pregnancies add up to a major nationwide effect. For the uninitiated who live outside the USA, the Super Bowl is the championship game of the US National Football League (NFL), played in late January or early February, attracting tens of millions of television viewers.

The study examined children who were born after, but conceived before, the Super Bowl, by mothers who lived no further than one county away from an NFL stadium, so mothers who were likely to be following their team as they made their way to the final, or part of a community doing this. The authors, Brian Duncan, Daniel Rees and Hani Mansour, used a sporting event for their study because these elicit intense emotions, but as they do not pollute the environment or threaten viewers with direct physical harm, or prevent access to antenatal care, they provide an opportunity to study the impact of 'pure' emotions on a pregnancy.

The study also found that so-called 'upset wins' (in other words where a team won who were not expected to, so their victory could not have been anticipated) are associated with larger increases in the probability of having a low-birth-weight child than are predicted wins, again suggesting it is the intensity of emotion the mother experiences during the pregnancy, as opposed to whether feelings are negative or positive, which is the central effect.

Petra Persson and Maya Rossin-Slater conclude their study[1] by pointing out that poorer women are subject to more stress than those who have more resources, so their results suggest that foetal stress exposure, given its negative impacts on their children, which endure even for decades into the future, may play a radical role in the intergenerational transmission of disadvantage.

While the current contagion of the virus is the focus of the world, it is also spreading stress and economic hardship, but maybe, behind the scenes, it is even consolidating inequality.

The mental health implications of the pandemic aren't just relevant to the current generation living through it; given this pregnancy research, which finds effects on the unborn, there are ominous and significant implications for the next generation being born now, or within nine months of the end of the pandemic. The adverse psychological impact appears to endure not just into the childhood of those being born now, but into their adulthood.

Is it possible that COVID-19 could extend its reach beyond the generation born during the pandemic? Could it reach even to the generation after that? In other words, the children of the children being born now or within the next nine months or so?

A study entitled 'Multigenerational effects of the 1918–19 influenza pandemic on educational attainment: Evidence from Sweden' used the Spanish Flu pandemic as a natural experiment to estimate the effects of a foetal health shock on the children of those who experienced the pandemic as a 'foetal insult'.[9] The study found that for women, the probability of higher education attendance drops by 3–5 percentage points if their mothers potentially experienced the Spanish Flu as a 'foetal insult'.[9] For men, the probability of attendance drops by 7–11 percentage points if their fathers were potentially prenatally exposed. The authors of the study conclude that the intergenerational consequences of prenatal health are much larger than previously imagined.

Is it also possible the pandemic could negatively impact future generations' psychology, beyond even the next epoch, maybe even the one after?

This is the startling conclusion of research published by a team of economists. Their study, entitled 'Epidemics and Trust: The Case of the Spanish Flu',[10] used measure of attitudes to trust in North Americans surveyed as adults from 1978 to 2018.

As part of an ongoing recurring survey across the United States involving a nationally representative large sample, one of the questions that is routinely asked is: 'Generally speaking, would you say that most people can be trusted or that you can't be too careful in dealing with people?'

The astonishing finding of this study is that experiencing the 1918–19 pandemic had permanent consequences in terms of individuals' social trust, even several generations later. Lower social trust was passed on to the descendants of the survivors of the Spanish Flu who migrated to the USA.

The Spanish Flu was by far the worst pandemic of modern times, infecting up to, depending on various estimates, either a third or maybe even 40 per cent of the entire world population. The result was an estimated 20 million – perhaps 50 million or even 100 million – deaths worldwide.

The authors argue that for the generation actually living through the Spanish Flu there were long-lasting frightening social consequences, leading naturally to a personal decline in trust in others. This resulted from having experienced massive social disruption and therefore generalised mistrust must itself have become pandemic as the influenza virus spread.

Countries that were neutral during the World War experienced less media and government censorship, so their populations endured coverage of the epidemic that was much more extensive, graphic and forthright. The authors of this study[10] argue that the specific lack of war censorship might have led these respective citizens to be more psychologically affected by the extent and severity of the pandemic. This would have adversely emotionally disturbed their social interactions accordingly. Consistent with this theory, the researchers did find a stronger reduction in social trust for the descendants of people migrating to the USA from countries heavily hit by the epidemic, yet which remained neutral during the war. The impact of the pandemic on trust was significantly worse in countries that remained neutral, not countries that were worse hit by the pandemic itself.

The researchers contend that this evidence suggests that less war coverage within these neutral countries, and in particular the specific lack of military censorship of the media, allowed citizens to more fully experience the extent and severity of the pandemic, and so alter their social interactions in a stronger way.

Experiencing the Spanish Flu and the associated social disruption with generalised mistrust had permanent consequences on individual behaviour. Individual social traits of higher levels of mistrust were then inherited by descendants. The authors argue their results are in line with other recent studies showing how large-scale crises impact individual psychology in a lasting way.

The very fact the pandemic is referred to as 'the Spanish Flu' is testament to the power of wartime censorship.[11] Spain was one of only a few major European countries to remain non-aligned during the First World War. Unlike those nations involved in armed conflict, where wartime censors suppressed news of the flu to avoid lowering morale, the Spanish media was unusually free to report on the epidemic in as much gruesome detail as they liked.

As a result, news of the influenza first hit the headlines in Madrid in late May 1918. Coverage moved up a gear after the Spanish King Alfonso XIII became infected. Since nations undergoing a press blackout could only read in-depth accounts from Spanish news sources, they naturally assumed that this was where the pandemic originated. The key difference lay not in the actual number of cases but more in Spain's neutrality, and therefore its lack of suppression of press coverage concerning the spread of the deadly disease. The Spanish themselves believed the virus had spread to them from France. They referred to it as the 'French Flu'.

With this historical context, tragic and stressful effects of COVID-19 unfortunately look likely to be passed down through generations.

22

WHAT HAPPENS IF THERE ARE NO DOCTORS?

If lockdown is like a general strike, what would happen if the doctors were also unavailable? What happens when doctors go on strike?

A national lockdown feels similar to a general strike.

The last time this happened in the UK was 4–12 May 1926, when over a million workers downed tools in solidarity with striking miners. This similarity was put to me by Dr Oliver Gloag during a podcast interview I was conducting on Camus' *The Plague*.

Oliver Gloag is an associate professor of French and Francophone studies at the University of North Carolina. I think he was suggesting this resemblance between a modern lockdown and an old-fashioned general strike because the absence of labour and services sharpens understanding over who we really need in our lives, and who we don't.

Those on the left of politics often support job walkouts, particularly general strikes, because they see an opportunity for the normally downtrodden workers to rediscover their real power. The grave danger, as indeed happened during the general strike in the 1920s, is that the economy adapts as people discover that services once deemed vital are in fact redundant. What actually occurred back then was that the government managed to mobilise enough backup resources (middle-class volunteers) to prevent the general strike becoming effective.

A strike can backfire, sometimes spectacularly. Can a lockdown?

Might we see a change in fundamental attitudes to what we think we need and want after the lockdown? Could the economy continue to suffer because large swathes of the population decide that a night out at the theatre, or at a swanky restaurant, is not money well spent? Might some habits of a lifetime now alter irreversibly? Or will there be a rebound effect? The 'roaring twenties' which followed the end of the last great planetary pandemic demonstrated a strong human need to make up for lost ground.

Might this, paradoxically, even apply to medicine, the one service that we seem to need most during a lockdown? Isn't that why we entered a lockdown in the first place? To 'save the health service'? Might the sacrifices required of the population lead to a fundamental reappraisal of just how important Western high-tech medicine is in our lives?

'Death is the enemy. But the enemy has superior forces. Eventually it wins.' *But does your doctor realise this?* The quoted lines are from Atul Gawande's book *Being Mortal: Medicine and What Matters in the End.*[1] The italics are my own. The full quote is:

> The simple view is that medicine exists to fight death and disease, and that is, of course, its most basic task. Death is the enemy. But the enemy has superior forces. Eventually, it wins. And, in a war that you cannot win, you don't want a general who fights to the point of total annihilation. You don't want Custer. You want Robert E. Lee, someone who knows how to fight for territory that can be won and how to surrender it when it can't, someone who understands that the damage is greatest if all you do is battle to the bitter end.

Before the pandemic, you only encountered a doctor offering medical advice in very particular circumstances, such as when you fell sick and attended an appointment in a clinic. Then, if they were properly trained, the medic would listen carefully to your account, examine you and run some tests, then offer a diagnosis and treatment plan that reflected not just your disease but also your personal physical and emotional characteristics.

You would have found it odd if you had attended an appointment and experienced the white-coated authority figure opposite you dispensing advice that was clearly tailored to someone else, not you. And yet there is a sense that this is exactly what has happened during the pandemic.

Prime ministers are flanked by chief medical officers who stare down the barrel of the TV lenses, and appear to be administering medical advice that is aimed specifically at you. What is really happening is very unusual: that doctor is acting as a physician to the nation, and treating the whole country as if it was their patient.

I am a strong believer in the power of Western scientific medicine. I trained in it and continue to see its supremacy over all other systems of knowledge about the body and mind when it comes to establishing the right diagnosis and therapeutics (usually, but not always).

Here is a quote from the now infamous cyclist Lance Armstrong which captures my sentiments:

> The night before brain surgery, I thought about death ... I asked myself what I believed ... I believed, too, in the doctors and the medicine and the surgeries – I believed in that. I believed in them. A person like Dr Einhorn [his oncologist], that's someone to believe in, I thought, a person with the mind to develop an experimental treatment twenty years ago that now could save my life. I believed in the hard currency of his intelligence and his research.[2]

Having said that, there are limits to medicine and medical knowledge. I believe that doctors should not just see patients but should also have the necessary wisdom to run hospitals. However, from that point onwards, I am less certain that medical knowledge should be the sole driver of decisions governing wider communities.

While I am convinced doctors should be in command of the operating theatre, I don't believe they should be in charge of the operation of a country. Yet this appears to be what has happened in many parts of the world. Politicians appear to have abrogated the responsibility of taking into account medical advice but balancing it against much wider considerations, such as liberty, the economy and even societal well-being.

The best way to ram home the message that medicine and health are way too important and complicated to be just left to the doctors, given the authority of physicians, is to examine what happens to people's health when doctors, en masse, leave the building. These are not conditions that tend to occur that often in wealthy countries, but in fact they do occur in certain situations, which allow the predicament to be scientifically studied.

When doctors strike, the scientific evidence finds that patients *stop* dying.

The most comprehensive review[3] of the medical impact of doctors' strikes is published in the prestigious academic journal *Social Science and Medicine*. A team led by Solveig Cunningham and Salim Yusuf at Emory and Georgetown Universities in the USA and McMaster University in Canada analysed five physician strikes around the world, all between 1976 and 2003. In the different strikes analysed, doctors withdrew their labour for between nine days and seventeen weeks. All the different studies report population mortality either stays the same, or even *decreases*, during medical strikes. Not a single study found death rates increased during the weeks of the strikes.

For example, in Los Angeles County, California, in January 1976, doctors went on strike in protest over soaring medical malpractice insurance premiums. For five weeks, approximately 50 per cent of doctors in the county reduced their practice and withheld care for anything but emergencies. One analysis, quoted by Cunningham and colleagues, found that the strike may have prevented more deaths than it caused.

It's the fact that elective, or non-emergency surgery, tends to stop during a doctors' strike, which seems to be the central factor. It looks like a surprising amount of mortality occurs following this kind of procedure, which disappears when elective surgery ceases as doctors withdraw their labour. Mortality declined steadily from the first week (21 deaths/100,000 population) to the sixth (13) and seventh (14), when mortality rates were lower than the averages of the previous five years. However, as soon as elective surgery resumed, there was a rise in deaths. There were ninety more deaths associated with surgery in the two weeks following the strike in 1976 (when doctors went back to work) than there had been during the same period in 1975.

Putting aside Los Angeles, what about the impact of doctors' industrial action where the majority of doctors participate, and the strike lasts several months?

Cunningham and colleagues[3] report on a strike in Jerusalem from 2 March to 26 June 1983 due to a salary dispute between the government and the Israel Medical Association; 8,000 of Jerusalem's 11,000 physicians refused to treat patients inside hospitals, though many of them set up separate aid stations where they treated emergency cases for a fee.

One analysis examined death certificates from several months surrounding the strike period, 16 February to 3 September 1983, and from a control period the previous year, 17 February to 3 September 1982. Mortality did not increase during or after the strike, even when elective surgery resumed. The pre-strike deaths for the control period and the strike period were identical at eighty-nine; there were six *fewer* deaths during the strike than during the control period, while in the ten weeks following the strike, there were seven more deaths than there had been in 1982.

In an intriguing example of how a doctors' strike can backfire, the authors of this particular mortality analysis argue that this apparent lack of impact of the strike on mortality suggests that there was an over-supply of doctors in Jerusalem at the time. The problem with drawing conclusions remains that the strike did not involve the wholescale deprivation of medical services.

Cunningham and colleagues point out in their review paper[3] that striking physicians opened aid stations, supplementing medical care and preventing people from mobbing the hospitals. While physicians were technically on strike during the four months of the dispute, most did not in fact adhere to the industrial action regulations. In truth, most doctors in Jerusalem provided care in a private or partially private context, so, while participating in spirit, they did not withdraw services.

Another intriguing study analysed changes in mortality by studying the *Jerusalem Post*'s newspaper reports of funerals during another Jerusalem doctors' strike, this time between March and June 2000. This one arose from the Israel Medical Association's conflict with the government's proposed salaries. The hospitals in the area cancelled all elective admissions and surgeries, but kept emergency rooms and other vital departments, such as dialysis units and oncology departments, open.

The funeral study found a *decline* in the number of funerals during the three months of the strike, compared with the same months of the previous three years. One burial society reported ninety-three funerals during one month of the strike (May 2000) compared with 153 in May 1999, 133 in May of 1998, and 139 in May 1997.

Cunningham and colleagues summarise their review of research assessing the effects of doctors' strikes on mortality, finding that four of the seven studies report mortality *dropped* as a result of medical industrial action, and three observed *no significant change* in mortality during the strike or in the period following.

There are several possible interpretations for this surprising finding. One is that as it's elective or non-emergency surgery which is usually most reduced in a doctors' strike, the mortality findings reflect this. The findings could be important because they could illuminate the relatively high risks of elective surgeries, which may increase mortality – a finding that perhaps would not have been highlighted if it wasn't for doctors' strikes.

Another sobering possible conclusion is that the public, and perhaps doctors themselves, overestimate the ability of medicine to stave off, or have an impact on, mortality. The problem with interpreting the data, as Cunningham and colleagues point out, is that in all medical strikes studied so far, not all doctors down tools.

Doctors' strikes don't necessarily drastically reduce access to healthcare. Given the purpose of most strikes is to deprive management of the workers' labour and its benefits, this raises the question of how effective a doctors' strike can ever be in comparison to other occupations. It is very difficult to get physicians to withdraw their labour. To be a doctor, the research on strikes illuminates, isn't an occupation, it's an identity. This issue of identity is why it's so much more difficult for doctors to strike. It's a characteristic prone to exploitation by governments and employers, frustrating standard union tactics.

Another theory as to why patients live longer when doctors go on strike is that the profession finally shakes off the shackles of its employer's restrictive practices, and returns, albeit temporarily, to practising medicine freely, as it would really like to. Perhaps – British Medical Association please take note – that's the most effective sort of industrial action doctors can ever take.

A recent study[4] published in the prestigious medical journal *Journal of the American Medical Association – Internal Medicine* found that high-risk patients with heart failure and cardiac arrest hospitalised in teaching hospitals experienced lower thirty-day mortality when admitted during dates of national cardiology professional or scientific meetings – when cardiologists are more likely to be out of town attending those conferences.

The authors of the study point out that in 2006, for example, nearly 19,000 cardiologists and other healthcare professionals attended the American Heart Association (AHA) annual meeting. A similar number of cardiologists and other professionals attend the American College of Cardiology (ACC) annual meetings.

During such conferences, physician staffing in hospitals is likely to be lower than on non-meeting dates, and the composition of physicians who remain to treat patients – rather than those who attend the meetings – may be different. These factors, one would have predicted, given it's likely that more senior doctors attend the prestigious conferences, may deleteriously affect treatment practices and outcomes for hospitalised patients.

Indeed, it is not an unusual gripe among junior colleagues that they feel they are forever 'covering' for senior physicians as they 'swan around' attending 'junkets' while the more junior members of the team are left to man the fort.

The study[4] was particularly interested in teaching hospitals because the authors hypothesised that mortality would be higher and treatment lower during cardiology meeting dates, and that these differences in outcomes would be largest in teaching hospitals, where a disproportionately larger fraction of cardiologists may attend cardiology conferences.

The authors conclude that mortality is lower among patients with high-risk of heart failure or cardiac arrest admitted to major teaching hospitals during the dates of national cardiology meetings. One explanation for this finding is that the intensity of care provided during meeting dates is 'lesser' and that for high-risk patients with cardiovascular disease, the harms of 'more' care may unexpectedly outweigh the benefits.

Another possible explanation, suggested by Ezekiel Emanuel writing in *The New York Times* about this study, is that while senior cardiologists are better researchers or academics, the junior physicians, fresher out of training, maybe more proficient clinically.

And yet another potential explanation, also suggested by Ezekiel Emanuel, is that senior cardiologists attempt more interventions. When the cardiologists were around, patients in cardiac arrest, for example, were significantly more likely to get intercessions, like stents, to open up their coronary blood vessels.

This study illuminates an uncomfortable possibility – that sometimes having a more senior doctor meddle in your care may be worse for your health.

Just in case some are tempted to dismiss this study of ten years of data involving tens of thousands of hospital admissions, there has been a similar investigation, this time in Japan, with not dissimilar results. This study[5] was entitled 'Is Survival After Out-of-Hospital Cardiac Arrests Worse During Days of National Academic Meetings in Japan? A Population-Based Study'. It looked at one-month survival with a neurologically favourable outcome after out-of-hospital cardiac arrests, which ought to be worse during days of national academic medical meetings because many medical professionals are then absent from clinics.

Calendar days at three national meetings (Japanese Society of Intensive Care Medicine, Japanese Association for Acute Medicine, and Japanese Circulation Society) were obtained for each year during the study period, because medical professionals who belong to these academic societies play an important role in treating out-of-hospital cardiac arrest patients after hospital admission.

The authors conclude that the proportion of patients with favourable neurological outcomes after cardiac arrests did not differ during academic medical meeting and non-meeting days. Indeed, there was a very small marginal benefit to having your cardiac arrest during the dates of these medical conferences when theoretically the top specialists would have been out of town.

While the debate will continue to rage over what these data mean, one recurring theme is that medicine and health are too complicated to be reduced to simple solutions or correlations, like that more doctors means better care, or that senior physicians are always better for patients than junior doctors. Good healthcare is about a lot more than just numbers of doctors or even their seniority. It requires a deeper analysis than that.

Where have we seen wisdom in this pandemic? The wisdom to take into account what the virologists, the epidemiologists, the physicians and also the economists and the philosophers have to say about the best way to balance health, well-being, liberty and the economy?

It is our politicians who are meant to be listening to the experts and then making decisions which take the evidence into account, but, critically, they must then synthesise a response which is not just a blind following of what they have been told.

Once you understand this problem, there can be no more terrifying a statement from a politician than '*We have been following the science...*'

23

CAN PANDEMIC PARANOIA PRODUCE MASS KILLING?

New research uncovers how pandemics and other catastrophes can drive us to war

Can the widespread emotional disturbance produced by a pandemic set off a cascade of psychological processes which inevitably result in armed conflict?

According to the psychology of 'scapegoating', the experience of profoundly negative shocks drives us to find others to blame. Harassment of scapegoats often begins as a result, eventually culminating in atrocities like holocausts and wars.

The 'Black Death' pandemic was the greatest decimation in European history. Forty per cent of the population died between 1347 and 1352; recent research into 'scapegoating' has illuminated the increased persecution of European Jews that followed.[1]

The bacterium which caused bubonic plague, or the 'Black Death', is *Yersinia pestis*, which was transmitted by fleas. Within less than a week, the bacteria spreads from the flea bite to the lymph nodes, producing the buboes, or swollen lumps, from which bubonic plague is named. The infection killed 70 per cent of its victims within ten days.

The need to find an enemy to blame during this cataclysm, according to some new academic research published in the academic *Journal of Economic Growth*, explains why Jews were tortured into confessing that they had initiated the plague by poisoning wells.

The results from the new study suggest that pandemics may ignite psychological processes which cause even more lethal atrocities later on. The 'Black Death' pandemic led to the largest massacres of Jews prior to the Holocaust; but the paranoia produced by the contagion may also have paved the way for the kind of anti-Semitism and scapegoating that underpinned future world wars and the Holocaust.

However, this investigation, published in 2019, also found that 'scapegoating' had not been inevitable wherever the Black Death had struck, suggesting that there must be ways of discouraging it. Entitled 'Negative Shocks and Mass Persecutions: Evidence from the Black Death', it found that the higher the level of mortality in a medieval European city, paradoxically the less likely it was that Jews would subsequently be persecuted there.

The authors have thereby uncovered a useful antidote to 'scapegoating': when people decide they need one another in order to survive a deadly crisis, then persecution goes down. Around one half of the cities with a Jewish community reported some form of persecution during the Black Death; however, the towns which experienced more severe plague outbreaks were less likely to persecute their Jewish community.

This might reflect the influence of the level of desperation upon the onset of persecution – which could be significant in predicting the impact of the COVID-19 outbreak in pushing us towards increased conflict and maybe even war.

An additional factor was that Jews were more likely to be victimised in towns where people were already more anti-Semitic. But cities that persecuted their Jewish community more during the Black Death grew more slowly in the following centuries, suggesting that 'scapegoating' is also generally an unproductive economic strategy. Jews were less likely to be abused – despite higher plague mortality rates – in cities where they offered specialised economic services, such as moneylending or trading.

The authors of the research conclude that the engagement of the minority and majority communities in economically mutually complementary activities may be a powerful way to reduce subsequent inter-group violence. Maybe we are less likely to hound the natives of the pandemic's country of origin if we still need them to provide ventilators, face masks and an airline industry. On the other hand, if the conspiracy theorists suspect them of having caused the pandemic because it served their economic interests – by virtue of having destroyed ours – then maybe future hostilities become that much more likely.

A huge role is played by the prevalence of pre-existing biases – be they cultural or economic – against the 'out-group' before the infection hits. Timing seems crucial. The cities that first experienced infection during a period when Christians were more disposed to blame Jews for the death of Jesus, for example over Easter, also experienced more persecution. The stage seems set for such violence when traditions exist, such as in medieval Toulouse, where members of the Jewish community were forced to pick one of their own every year to be publicly slapped in the face on Good Friday.[1]

Another recent paper, 'Do Natural Disasters Enhance Societal Trust?',[2] examined 3,799 disaster events from 105 countries over the 1970–2000 period and found that it was similarly easy to predict whether or not people bonded together in the face of community collapse. The study argues that while some naturally occurring disasters such as storms can have devastating human and economic impacts, nevertheless an unexpected social benefit of greater 'hurricane' exposure appears to be a more tightly knit society. Some natural disasters provide the opportunity for societies to bond by working closely together to meet their collective challenges.

Whether people collect together as opposed to fracturing and fighting one another may depend on the kind of catastrophe they face. Disasters which tend to have widely differing effects on the rich as compared with the poor, such as floods (poorer groups are usually much more highly exposed), erode social networks and trust. On the other hand, some types of disasters – for example, storms – affect social classes more uniformly, generating greater cooperation across communities. This study confirms that floods increase distrust in a country, while storms improve trust.

A contagious disease targets people and leaves buildings intact, and this may predispose a population to becoming even more paranoid that this may have been part of some enemy conspiracy, even a bio-weapon. It also means that congregational acts like repairing a bridge or church are less likely to happen, and therefore public acts of solidarity become less tangible, meaning less of the necessary social cohesion.

Was the rapid spread of an 'epidemic' of public clapping for healthcare staff at appointed hours across Europe a good example of this? It was a moving act of solidarity, yet it also seemed somewhat feeble. If neighbours were allowed to bond together and do something more practically helpful, maybe this would build community solidarity more effectively and inoculate against scapegoating. But blanket social distancing has the inadvertent effect of preventing this.

The random acts of solidarity on display in the midst of this pandemic appear somewhat chance and haphazard. Maybe there should even be teams tasked with creating these kinds of bonding events in every locale, given the challenges of social distancing?

The powerful psychological motives to scapegoat are so strong, however, that clumsy official interventions could make things even worse. For example, the Italian press had accused Russia of secreting military spies among a group of doctors dispatched to the centre of Italy's coronavirus epidemic.[3] President Vladimir Putin apparently offered to help during a phone call with Prime Minister Giuseppe Conte. Moscow then gifted nine aircraft and more than 100 experts, along with medical supplies, to Milan.

Italian sources now claim that 80 per cent of the aid was useless. The delivery, therefore, began to appear more like a 'pretext'. Instead it is now claimed that Russia's 104-strong aid contingent, run by the military, contained intelligence operatives.

The Russian Embassy in Rome tweeted a condemnation of the Italian press for 'Russophobic Cold War fake news'. The war of words escalated between Italy and Russia, which betrays another reason our leaders may have a very powerful vested interest in encouraging 'scapegoating'.

Historically, politicians have positively encouraged scapegoating because it helps distract an electorate from blaming their own government for the chaos produced by a pandemic. Instead, scapegoating produces a target-rich environment of external enemies. This confusion conveniently diverts attention away from the enemy within, which is our administration's own incompetence.

The virus invades our own cells and hijacks them to reproduce and spread; but the psychology of the pandemic indicates that powerful emotions can be similarly hijacked and diverted to ignite wars and pogroms, which then devastate just as much as the disease.[4] The research reported here demonstrates there is a way to understand history so we can inoculate ourselves against repeating it.[4]

The life-saving arrival of vaccines might yet backfire. Witness the increasing conflict between competing nations, desperate to get hold of them, intent on depriving other countries, in the ensuing scramble.

How long before the growing tensions between communities and governments, unchecked by the rapid injection of a mental vaccine that promotes teamwork as the better answer, erupt into armed conflict?[5]

24

DOES FIGHTING COVID ON THE STREETS NEED A NEW CHURCHILL?

How crucial is inspiration if we are to survive?

As the world faced an unprecedented crisis, where were the stirring speeches that would keep us inspired to keep fighting on, no matter what our government or the coronavirus threw at us?

Gary Oldman won the Best Actor Oscar for his portrayal of Winston Churchill in the movie *Darkest Hour*, and had apparently been inspiring standing ovations in cinemas on both sides of the Atlantic after delivering Churchill's famous lines.[1] The film was nominated for a Best Picture Oscar as well. Is there a particular psychology to the inspiration of Churchill's speeches which might explain the film's success, and, rather more importantly, British victory in a war it seemed destined to lose? If so, where does the psychological power of a great speech come from?

Don't we all need inspiration at times of personal and national crisis? For example, how many of us are deeply bored by lifeless jobs and uninspiring bosses? A tough pep talk to demotivated employees is the centrepiece of the award-winning film *Glengarry Glen Ross*. Failing real-estate salesmen receive a motivational kick from Alec Baldwin in an infamous 'Always Be Closing' speech:

> Get mad you son of a bitches, get mad. You want to know what it takes to sell real estate? It takes BRASS BALLS to sell real estate. Go

and do likewise, gents. Money's out there. You pick it up, it's yours. You don't, I got no sympathy for you...

Did Michael Douglas achieve the Oscar for Best Actor in *Wall Street* partly because of his 'Greed is Good' speech?

The point is, ladies and gentleman, that greed, for lack of a better word, is good. Greed is right, greed works. Greed clarifies, cuts through, and captures the essence of the evolutionary spirit. Greed, in all of its forms; greed for life, for money, for love, knowledge has marked the upward surge of mankind. And greed, you mark my words, will not only save Teldar Paper, but that other malfunctioning corporation called the USA. Thank you very much.

Soldiers whose courage is wavering need a rousing talk from generals, just like Russell Crowe's call to arms in the movie *Gladiator:*

My name is Maximus Decimus Meridius, Commander of the Armies of the North, General of the Felix Legions, loyal servant to the true emperor, Marcus Aurelius. Father to a murdered son, husband to a murdered wife. And I will have my vengeance, in this life or the next.

Does the psychology of such an inspirational speech also explain why the film scooped Best Picture, Best Actor for Crowe and three other Oscars?

Athletes need encouraging, which is why a stirring speech from the coach is such a recurrent feature in sports films. The famous 'Inches Speech' by Al Pacino's coach in the movie *Any Given Sunday*, imploring his football players to sacrifice for one another, might move a cinema audience, but would it motivate you in real life?

This was tested scientifically in a psychology study[2] entitled 'The Influence of a Simulated "Pep Talk" on Athlete Inspiration, Situational Motivation, and Emotion', where 151 actual college football players were randomly assigned to watch this inspirational four-minute half-time speech, or viewed a clip from the same movie in which mundane game instructions are issued by the same coach.

The research found those players who watched Al Pacino calling his players to come together and take the game 'inch by inch' were more inspired to perform and were imbued with greater emotional dominance. The authors point out that, given the particular psychological characteristics of American college football, dominance might be imperative.

Robert Steele, a psychologist at Wesleyan University in the USA, specifically investigated the psychological impact of Churchill's speeches and found that listening to an actor reading excerpts of just seven minutes from Winston Churchill's speech on Dunkirk produced significant psychological changes in listeners. 'Power motivation, activation, and inspirational speeches'[3] found that listening to Churchill made people feel significantly more powerful and with added desire to be active. Robert Steele had previously investigated the psychological power of inspirational speeches, finding they even released significantly higher levels of adrenaline in the body.

Psychologists Todd Thrash and Andrew Elliot[4] found that how inspired you are plays a significant role in everyday well-being. For example, inspiration levels predict how absorbed you are at work, higher self-esteem and more optimism about your future. Their study, published in the *Journal of Personality and Social Psychology*, suggests we may harbour a deep psychological need for inspiration, perhaps in particular at times of crisis. For example, the study cites evidence that cancer patients prefer contact with other patients who are doing better than they are. It's not enough to talk the talk, you have to walk the walk as well: these cancer patients were inspiring because of what they had endured.

Andrew Bowman's study[5] 'The Mantle of the Prophet: Churchill's Embodiment of the Prophetic Ethos' points out that prophets have a particular grip on us in their journey from the wilderness, and given his political unpopularity before the war, Churchill's career echoes that of the prophet who has to first endure being outcast, as he had been from his party.

Bowman points out that when Churchill became prime minister, there was no evidence that Britain could win a war with Germany. The German army had swept across Europe, and looked unbeatable. It took the inspirational Churchill to confound expectations by announcing with certainty that Britain would defeat Germany, yet he had no evidence to support his assertion. But he could reliably invoke strong emotions in his listeners through charismatic speeches.

Can we scientifically analyse a speech to uncover what is the secret behind inspiration, and then deploy the finding to assist us in our own lives?

The most memorable and inspirational political speeches of the past century, including Martin Luther King Jr's 'I have a dream' oration and Winston Churchill's 'iron curtain' declamation, are built on metaphors. This is the argument of a study entitled 'Presidential leadership and charisma: The effects of metaphor',[6] measuring the incidence of metaphors in first-term inaugural addresses of thirty-six US presidents. Presidents found to be more charismatic used nearly twice as many metaphors as non-charismatic presidents. The authors of the study argue that metaphors are inspiring because they stir up emotional connections while also conveying the message of action.

Churchill may even have persuaded the USA to enter the war with his powerful metaphor of the UK needing rescuing as the two countries were 'travelling companions'. Churchill's speeches inspired victory because they transformed the way the USA thought about Britain, and the way the British thought about their resilience, and their place in the world.

That's the kind of inspiration we all need when we're in crisis.

Research by Mary Helen Immordino-Yang and Lesley Sylvan[7] leads these two neuroscientists to suggest that admiring others, and being inspired by them, could be fundamental to motivating us. Their study argues that admiration for another person's virtue stimulates a desire to be virtuous ourselves, and encourages us to strive to overcome odds that would normally defeat us.

The problem, however, is that if we suffer from low self-esteem, or feel life has been unfair to us, we tend to view others who are achieving something we ourselves are struggling with – like losing weight or passing an exam – with envy, and we tend to denigrate their achievements. We often feel they have unfair advantages over us.

This acts to prevent us deriving the necessary motivational impetus we might otherwise gain from admiring the achievements of others and being inspired by their 'virtue'. Virtue itself is an interesting concept, given that the ancient Greeks were preoccupied with what it was to lead the virtuous life; whereas today we seem more bothered with competing with our neighbours and getting ahead, rather than being ourselves the source of inspiration to others.

In their study, entitled 'Admiration for Virtue: Neuroscientific perspectives on a motivating emotion',[7] these researchers started by wondering if admiration for the virtuous behaviour of others was a somewhat abstract emotion, and would therefore not have the power to galvanise the kind of basic physiological preparedness we often see stoked up in, for example, a fight-or-flight scenario. In such a situation, strong emotions – most often terror – get our heart pumping and other systems are brought online to get us to perhaps the most highly motivated state there is – to defend or run in order to save our lives.

This research started with a question: if the emotion of admiration for virtue could be induced experimentally in the laboratory, would the neuroscientists also see the activation of similar fight-or-flight systems in the brain and brain stem that maintain basic survival and prepare the body for action? These would include such powerful systems as those that modulate heart rate, blood pressure, and hormones.

In their study, they put subjects inside a brain scanner which would monitor how brain activity responds to true stories of enormous courage and overcoming adversity (designed to provoke admiration for virtue), while they also measured heart and respiration rate changes.

In one true story used in the study, a young blind German woman, despite all odds, learns fluent Tibetan by ear, invents a computerized Tibetan Braille system to translate texts, and travels into the mountains of Tibet to open a school for blind children, to which she dedicates her life.

The researchers were particularly interested in what changes might occur in particular parts of the brain we already know are associated with strong emotion and therefore theoretically powerful motivation. For example, we know that a brain region referred to as the anterior insula 'feels' the inside of the body, allowing us to experience a stomach ache or a racing heartbeat. This part of the brain has also been associated with the process of feeling emotion-related transformations in the body, such as the 'punched-in-the-gut' feeling associated with learning bad news, or the sense of revulsion associated with unfair decisions.

The study found that activation in the anterior insular cortex involved in feeling these bodily changes began on average four to six seconds later in the emotion process when hearing admirable stories of virtue, and was subsequently sustained. In contrast, activation in this area during less complex emotions unrelated to meaningful motivation, like empathy for another person's misfortune, happened almost immediately and died down relatively quickly, on average after a few seconds.

What this study suggests is that admiration for virtue in others could be an underestimated powerful emotion. It could therefore be harnessed to help motivate us to achieve difficult tasks requiring sustained tenacity, such as losing weight or passing arduous exams.

The problem is that, often, if we take the example of losing weight, we feel negative emotions such as envy and resentment towards those who are fitter and look better than us, rather than using these examples to motivate us by focusing on admiration for the virtue being demonstrated.

This kind of research suggests we should look around us and more clearly see the virtue in those we meet and who might therefore be harnessed as examples that could motivate us.

If we ignore admiration for virtue, we are neglecting an indispensable motivational strategy that could enhance our lives.

There was something about the elderly, frail Captain Sir Tom Moore struggling up and down his garden to raise money for NHS charities which was clearly inspirational to the nation. But his actions also ignited trolling, as we saw in a previous chapter, suggesting the very act which inspires some upsets others.

25

THE 'BOOMERANG' EFFECT OF VACCINATING THREE FORMER US PRESIDENTS

'Boomerang' effect psychology explains why health campaigns can backfire

Three former US presidents – Barack Obama, Bill Clinton and George W. Bush – agreed to be recorded and broadcast taking the COVID-19 vaccine.[1] It's just the first of perhaps many dramatic attempts to encourage the public to be vaccinated. This stunt is supposed to persuade or inspire us to get vaccinated too; but why should this be the effect, and is it possible that this strategy might backfire?

Obama was quoted in *The Guardian:* 'I may end up taking it on TV or having it filmed, just so that people know that I trust this science.' George W. Bush's chief of staff told CNN that the former president was prepared to take the vaccine on camera 'to help encourage his fellow citizens to get vaccinated'. Clinton's press secretary also revealed that he too was set to be videoed as he receives the vaccine, explaining he would do it in a public setting 'if it will help urge all Americans to do the same'.

These are supposedly high-credibility individuals; why would they endanger their own lives if the vaccine was dicey? The public relations strategy behind the frenetic push to get the vaccine accepted could not be more obvious. But do these proposed media stunts in fact reveal mounting anxiety that not enough people will agree to be vaccinated, so prolonging the pandemic?

Now that a vaccine is here, it may be that the major barrier is getting enough of the population to take it. Why is that so important? Have we not already overcome the biggest hurdle to killing COVID-19 – achieving an effective vaccine? From now on in, surely life is going to get easier?

It turns out that if you want to end an epidemic, how effective a vaccine is becomes less important than the number of people taking it up.

A new study from the Yale School of Public Health and Harvard Medical School used a mathematical simulation of vaccination and discovered that implementation contributed much more to the success of vaccination programs compared with a vaccine's effectiveness. The investigation, entitled 'Clinical Outcomes Of A COVID-19 Vaccine: Implementation Over Efficacy',[2] found that the benefits of a vaccine decline considerably in the face of manufacturing or deployment delays, or substantial vaccine hesitancy. A poll by Gallup, as reported in *The Guardian* and released in mid-November, revealed that in the USA, 42 per cent of the population would not take the vaccine, even if it was 'available right now at no cost'.

So will the impact of three former US presidents being vaccinated, and similar publicity stunts, where we are machine-gunned with image after image of public figures being vaccinated, deliver?

Psychologists who have studied overcoming public resistance in similar predicaments have uncovered a famous 'boomerang' effect: the tendency for public health campaigns to spectacularly backfire and produce the opposite outcome to that intended.

A study entitled 'Government Health Warnings and the "Boomerang" Effect',[3] for example, found that the old-fashioned written government health warning on cigarette advertisements can indeed 'boomerang'. The research established that health warnings in cigarette advertising increased the desire to smoke, with the amplified yearning even greater for smokers than for non-smokers.

There has been a shift in recent years to deploying graphic imagery on cigarette packets, including vivid pictures of diseased lungs and mouths, people dying of lung cancer, and even corpses. Yet these tactics too have been found to backfire. A study[4] from a team at the University of Illinois found using graphic imagery on cigarette packets resulted in unintended effects, potentially wrecking the intended message. A significant number of people felt their sense of freedom was threatened, with increased negative perceptions of the source as domineering, along with more anger as well.

As we value freedom and choice (perhaps particularly in the USA and maybe the wider Western world), dogmatic, explicit or forceful messages might arouse an emotional reaction against them, particularly if we feel our autonomy is threatened. Maybe it was this psychological thinking which lay behind President-elect Joe Biden announcing Americans won't be forced to take a vaccine.

Far Eastern societies such as South Korea, China and Taiwan demonstrated much better results compared to the West on all counts earlier in the pandemic, perhaps because their citizenry was more willing to give up freedoms; so test and tracing, as well lockdowns, were more comprehensive in these nations.

As vaccinating gets rolled out across the world, a widening chasm in outcomes might be revealed for such cultural reasons. Vaccines could then widen the gap in economic and health performance between advanced capitalist societies in the East and the West.

Researchers Aharon Levy and Yossi Maaravic[5] account for the 'boomerang' effect by invoking the notion we are all driven by powerful, innate needs to preserve a positive self-image. When confronted with information that our prior beliefs were wrong, this threatens the self-image we want to project – that we are consistent, reasonable and rational people. Their study, 'The boomerang effect of psychological interventions', concludes that this psychological background means we become energised to justify our beliefs even more strongly, so resisting change. To adopt the new opposing position has negative connotations for the public image we wish to maintain.

The worrying thing that the mass immunisation strategy against Covid seems to be in grave danger of missing is that attitudes to vaccination are often central to people's sense of themselves; attacking them may backfire.

'Populist politics and vaccine hesitancy in Western Europe: An analysis of national-level data'[6] found a highly significant positive association between the percentage of people in a country who voted for populist parties and the proportion who believe that vaccines are neither important nor effective. Populists seek to divide the world into masses and elites, claiming to represent the former while opposing the latter.

The study also found there was a similar association between populist party support and the percentage of people who think vaccines are unsafe, but it wasn't quite as strong as the other two associations.

Author Jonathan Kennedy[6] concludes that vaccine hesitancy and political populism may be driven by similar psychological forces: a profound distrust of elites and experts. Using elites to ram home your message – and you can't get more elite than three former US presidents – may therefore backfire. The vaccination strategy might 'boomerang', relying as it does on experts to originate the tactics.

Maybe this is because these very authorities have themselves never been more psychologically quarantined from the population they are trying to inoculate.

26

COVID ON THE COUCH: SIGMUND FREUD'S SURPRISING ANALYSIS

What would the founder of psychoanalysis, Sigmund Freud, say today about coping?

In classical psychoanalysis, as pioneered by Sigmund Freud (1856–1939), the patient reclines on a couch while the therapist sits *behind* them, and so cannot be seen directly by the client.

Freud advocated that the clinical encounter should not be 'face-to-face'. Was this an early attempt at 'social distancing'? Sigmund Freud did, after all, live through the Spanish Flu pandemic of 1918–20.

Meeting in a consulting room, but then deploying a furniture arrangement which on purpose 'hides' the psychoanalyst from the patient, according to Freud, generates powerful psychological processes. This setup supposedly encouraged patients to recount whatever came to mind without censoring themselves. Otherwise, if they could see the therapist frown as they began disclosing, this might inhibit revelation.

Have you noticed how a much more intimate conversation sometimes evolves when you are sitting *next* to someone, in a car for example, so not looking directly at them?

During the current pandemic, social distancing rules mean that therapists can't physically meet with patients. What are the implications for the more 'hardcore' or 'old-fashioned' psychoanalysis, as established by Sigmund Freud, where the patient doesn't see you directly but is in the same room with you? How can that be replicated with remote working?

The International Psychoanalytic Association has published some guidance on its website:[1]

> Some patients that lie down on a couch might prefer not to see the analyst during the remote session. They can do this by turning off the video option or by placing the device/video screen in a position in which they cannot see it. The risk of doing this is that if the connection suddenly fails, the patient may not be aware of this situation and will continue talking.

In the UK's *The Guardian* of 23 April 2020, psychotherapist Gary Greenberg published an article entitled 'Therapy Under Lockdown – I'm just as terrified as my patients are'.[2]

He describes how using a laptop to conduct the sessions 'face-to-face' introduces new challenges for the therapist. These include being able to see inside, into the patient's home for the first time. Will whatever is glimpsed over the patient's shoulder now distract the psychoanalyst? Among many difficulties that Gary Greenberg confesses, he notes that Sigmund Freud, the father of psychoanalysis, and therefore the originator of modern psychotherapy as we understand it, didn't appear to offer that much help in this current pandemic predicament:

> Freud placed his bet on the human, as the source of both suffering and balm. He didn't reckon with a nemesis so indifferent as a virus, any more than he worried about a meteor crashing into the Earth or the sun suddenly being snuffed out … we are stuck with the imperative to restrain ourselves to a degree that Freud did not anticipate … At a time when we need each other badly, when we are under attack not by human nature but by nature itself, the best we can do to take care of one another is to stay away from one another. Even Freud at his most misanthropic never imagined that… Perhaps this is not the time to ask 'What would Sigmund do?' He's not much of a role model in normal times, let alone times like these…

Is it really true that Freud 'didn't reckon with a nemesis so indifferent as a virus'?

The last great viral pandemic that the Western world faced before the current one was the 1918 Spanish Flu pandemic. Freud's daughter,

Sophie Halberstadt-Freud, died from the Spanish Flu in 1920. She was twenty-seven years old.

Peculiarly, mortality during the 1918 pandemic peaked at the exact age of twenty-eight, in other words young people in their late twenties were oddly vulnerable to that virus.

One theory, described in a paper entitled 'Age-Specific Mortality During the 1918 Influenza Pandemic: Unravelling the Mystery of High Young Adult Mortality',[3] whose lead author was Alain Gagnon, a demographer at the University of Montreal, is that this generation had been exposed to the so-called Russian Flu, which was a pandemic of the early 1890s, just after being born. Alain Gagnon has argued that it might be that exposure to a previous viral infection at a particular early age may somehow prime the body, which then reacts especially badly to another infection later in life. This theory is now being investigated to see if it explains why it is now older adults, not those in their early twenties, who appear particularly vulnerable to COVID-19.

Given what we know now about the vulnerability of an older age group to this coronavirus, Gagnon wrote somewhat prophetically back in 2013: 'Knowledge of the age-pattern of susceptibility to mortality from influenza could improve crisis management during future influenza pandemics.'[3]

While the jury is still out on that particular theory, we continue to be bombarded with a plethora of scientific answers to the modern plague, so it is tempting to also turn to psychiatric 'science' for the solution to our mental suffering.

What did Freud do? How did he cope before the advent of all the modern scientific advances in psychiatry and psychology? What was his response to dealing with bereavement in the middle of a pandemic?

Freud wrote a letter to Oskar Pfister on 27 January 1920, just two days after the death of his beloved daughter:

This afternoon we received the news that our sweet Sophie in Hamburg had been snatched away by influenzal pneumonia, snatched away in the midst of glowing health, from a full and active life as a competent mother and loving wife, all in four or five days, as though she had never existed. Although we had been worried about her for a couple of days, we had nevertheless been hopeful; it is so difficult to judge from a distance. And this distance must remain distance; we were not able to travel at once, as we had intended, after the first alarming news; there was no train, not even for an emergency. The undisguised brutality of our time is weighing heavily upon us. Tomorrow she is to be cremated, our poor Sunday child!... Sophie leaves two sons, one of six, the other thirteen months, and an inconsolable husband who will have to pay dearly for the happiness of these seven years. The happiness existed exclusively within them; outwardly there was war, conscription, wounds, the depletion of their resources, but they had remained courageous and gay.[4]

It is also in a previous letter[5] to Pfister, a priest and a psychotherapist, dated 10 September 1918, that Freud makes a revelation about his view of human nature, which is one of his most infamous quotes: 'I do not break my head very much about good and evil, but I have found little that is "good" about human beings on the whole. In my experience most of them are trash.'[5]

In the end, did his own suffering, and that he experienced in his patients, embitter Freud?

The psychiatrist Anthony Storr, in his book *Freud: A Very Short Introduction*, explains that

... in his clinical work Freud was kind and tolerant ... however his kindness was not based on any great expectations of the human race, whom he regarded with distaste or with detachment rather than with love.[6]

Anthony Storr concludes:

Where human frailty was concerned, Freud exhibited a quite unusual tolerance. This, because it has led to a more civilized attitude towards neurosis, sexual deviation, and other forms of emotional maladaptation, is one of Freud's most valuable legacies...

Freud never believed that advances in science, particularly neuroscience, would ultimately provide an answer to the problem of human suffering.[7] Instead, the solution would arise out of the way we treated each other, and our understanding of ourselves and our emotions. There was a sense in which he believed this was forever beyond the reach of laboratory experiments.

Maybe one reason why some are not finding psychotherapy so helpful is that modern treatment has for too long over-emphasised technique, theory and academic teaching, at the expense of the human.

The real legacy of Freud that might be most valuable right now comes through his humanity when directly confronting the reality of human suffering.[8]

On 11 April 1929, Sigmund Freud wrote to his friend the psychiatrist Ludwig Binswanger, who was grieving for the death of his eldest son, Robert, at just twenty years old:

> My daughter who died would have been thirty-six today ... We know that the acute sorrow we feel after such a loss will run its course, but also that we will remain inconsolable, and will never find a substitute. No matter what may come to take its place, even should it fill that place completely, it remains something else. And that is how it should be. It is the only way of perpetuating a love that we do not want to abandon.[9]

EPILOGUE

Spreading the story of the science of survival

All things come to an end – including, eventually, pandemics. The virus doesn't just destroy lives and livelihoods: there was also an epidemic of unexpected emotional effects. Notably, COVID-19 appeared to unleash a tsunami of apathy, even as it evoked unprecedented heroism and neighbourly solidarity.

It is the psychology of the phenomenon which has been mostly neglected, or ignored, or avoided. The contagion held up a brutal mirror for all to stare into.

For the first time in recent history, because of lockdown, we were prevented from indulging in all those distractions with which we had traditionally filled our lives, and which also divert us from truly examining ourselves. Left with nothing else to do, we were faced with absolutely no alternative but to stare into this reflection, and see only ourselves glowering back. Stripped of everything that cluttered our existence, it was not a pretty picture.

It turned out that while some valiantly struggled on regardless of the obstacles the virus placed in their way, others used the pandemic as an endless excuse for not doing their bit. To survive we have to learn the correct lessons; but it's still not clear we will, nor will our governments – particularly if we continue to deny the psychology of our predicament.

The statistics over infection rates, death numbers and hospital admissions have dominated the news and policy-making. Just because mental and emotional health are neither as measurable, nor as visible, does not mean these areas of profound impact should be ignored in the way they have been.

If you agree with the alternative message of practical hope in these pages, I trust that you will also try to spread the story of the science of survival that I want you to have found here. We need to roll out this psychological vaccine. And we need to do it urgently, because the pandemic continues to be cruel, random and deeply unjust and we are running out of time to protect ourselves from profound impacts which will persist across generations.

The impacts on pregnancy during a pandemic, as well as other effects, could have ramifications which endure for decades to come. Just as inoculation against the various viruses involved will probably have to be tweaked to deal with all the evolving variants, resilience requires us to learn the flexibility required to adapt to new stresses and strains.

This is the mental vaccine. In a pandemic of COVID-19, and in life from now on, things can never be the same again.

Survival is possible. But survival is also a decision. Endurance may require a fundamental re-think about many of the foundations which we previously took for granted, about what life was about.

We build resilience by transforming our lives so we can keep going – no matter how long this new state of affairs is to last – as opposed to trying to muddle through, crossing our fingers, banking on an end sometime soon. I believe I have provided enough evidence for you to question many of the assumptions on which official advice on surviving the pandemic has been based.

You may recall, right back at the beginning of our encounter, the example we cited of Meghan and Harry's advice, in their first podcast, that 'love always wins'. It was this banality which inspired us to attempt to distill a more practically helpful Mental Vaccine for Covid-19.

But a lot happened between Meghan and Harry's first podcast, at the start of 2021, and 'that' interview they gave to Oprah Winfrey on 7 March 2021. How does that 'love always wins' advice stack up now, given Meghan's new startling confession of falling so low as to become suicidal?

The media and the public seemed, in fact, by the time of the interview, to have completely forgotten the 'love always wins' sentiment; but then again, practically all the advice on emotional health dispensed during the pandemic appeared equally forgettable.

Also, another problem the media and public appeared to miss is that in discussing suicide so openly during an Oprah Winfrey interview, might she in fact have made it more likely that others will self-harm? In attempting to confront these serious mental health issues more directly than has hitherto been done, do we run the same risk?

Are Meghan, Harry or Oprah Winfrey aware that media reporting of suicidal behaviour has been found to contribute to an increase in suicidal thinking and actual suicides in the population?[1]

Google searches for 'How to kill yourself' significantly increased after the release of *13 Reasons Why*, a popular American teen drama on the aftermath of a high school student's suicide. The study[2] calculated there were 900 000 to 1.5 million more searches than expected for that time of year in just over two weeks following the release of the series.

Another study,[3] published in the *Journal of the American Academy of Child & Adolescent Psychiatry* in February 2020, estimated there were 195 additional suicide deaths among ten- to seventeen-year-old youths between 1 April and 31 December 2017, following the show's release.

The suicide of actress Marilyn Monroe was associated with a 12 per cent increase in suicide.[1] Publicity surrounding the death of the comedic actor Robin Williams was linked with an increase of more than 1,800 deaths in the United States in late 2014.[4]

However, new research suggests that, in fact, in talking about suicide, Meghan Markle may have indeed performed a positive service for suicide prevention.

The study[5] refers to a 'Papageno Effect', which the authors claim happens when suicide rates go down following a particular kind of self-harm publicity.

The 'Papageno Effect' is based on Papageno's overcoming of a suicidal crisis in Mozart's opera *The Magic Flute*. If media reporting has a preventive impact this should now be referred to as the 'Papageno Effect', the authors argue.[5] In the opera, Papageno becomes suicidal upon fearing the loss of his beloved Papagena; however, he refrains from suicide because of three boys who draw his attention to alternative coping strategies.[5]

Thomas Niederkrotenthaler and Gernot Sonneck from the Medical University of Vienna, Austria, led a team who analysed all 497 suicide-related print media reports from the eleven largest Austrian nationwide newspapers including the term 'suicide' between 1 January and 30 June 2005.[5]

Reporting of individuals thinking about suicide (not accompanied by attempted or completed suicide) was associated with a decrease in national suicide rates.[5] This study suggests that media items on suicidal thinking, perhaps as described by Meghan in her recent interview, formed a distinctive class of articles which have a low probability of being potentially harmful, and might instead be helpful.

The authors conclude that the actual reporting of suicidal thinking may contribute to preventing suicide. Therefore, it follows that whatever Piers Morgan may think or believe about the Meghan interview, the latest scientific research suggests she may have performed a public service in drawing attention to suicidal thinking.

One theory as to why this might be the case is that news of someone surviving suicidal impulses may enhance audience identification with the reported individual, and thus highlights the reported outcome as 'going on living'.[5]

This research suggests a new public health strategy as regards suicide prevention. This may be most effective when articles are published on individuals who refrained from adopting suicidal plans, and instead adopted positive coping mechanisms, despite suffering adverse circumstances.

The authors refer to this kind of press story as 'Mastery of Crisis'.[5] One example they quote: 'Before [Tom Jones] had his first hit, he thought about suicide … and wanted to jump in front of an Underground train in London … In 1965, before he made the charts with "It's not unusual", he thought for a second: "If I just take a step to the right, then it'll all be over."'

Whatever else you may think of her, or the interview, the key question becomes, did Meghan exhibit 'Mastery Of Crisis'?

Part of the deeper psychological reason why Meghan's interview with Oprah provoked such controversy was, perhaps, many found it hard to believe the privileged could end up suffering such emotional torment. Yet any of us can find ourselves living inside a kind of mental prison, no matter how transparent the walls may seem to the outside world.

Did the pandemic not become a prison in many different ways?

But catastrophic life events, from bad marriages to bullying at school, also are torments that derive their particular pain from rendering us feeling trapped. At a psychological level, maybe this is partly why there is a whole genre of movies based on prisons: their unconscious emotional appeal is that we all feel incarcerated from time to time.

Indeed, *The Shawshank Redemption*, the number one rated movie of all time according to users of the Internet Movie Database,[6] is set inside a prison. Perhaps surprisingly for such a popular film, the plot features two completed as well as two attempted suicides.

In a sobering lesson for those who believe that ending lockdown and the pandemic will lead to similar relief in mental health problems, the first suicide in the movie occurs after a long-term inmate is released. Brooks finds it too difficult to cope with life outside of the cloistered conditions he had become used to over five decades on the inside.[6]

He eventually writes a letter to his friends: 'I don't like it here. I'm tired of being afraid all the time. I've decided not to stay'. He desperately carves 'Brooks was here' into a wood ceiling beam and then hangs himself from it.

But, in the face of multiple set-backs, including the blow of hearing about the death of Brooks, the hero of the film, Andy, declares: 'I guess it comes down to a simple choice, really. Get busy living or get busy dying.'[6]

I won't spoil the end of the film for those who haven't seen it, but suffice it to say that Andy refuses, right from the beginning of his internment, to be contained by any physical prison. Instead, he relentlessly seeks mental liberation from every constraint placed on his life.

The pandemic became a kind of prison, but emotional breakout was possible: you just needed effective mental tunnelling equipment. Without it, breakdown was inevitable.

As you finish the course of treatment that is the Mental Vaccine for COVID-19, and as we finally put the kit away, where was sharpest point of our needle? Maybe, arguably, it was the vital importance of locating places of emotional safety during these hazardous times. This is the first of the many practical steps we advocated to assist you in mastering the crisis.

A lot of the trouble many got into was that the strain of the pandemic meant they became psychologically disturbed, meaning their 'place of safety' ended up being actually rather dangerous.

On 6 February 2021, Chris Lewis, sixty, was part of the Patterdale Mountain Rescue Team called out on an emergency rescue to Red Screes above Kirkstone Pass in the Lake District.[7] Two men had travelled from Liverpool and Leicester to camp overnight in that wilderness. As reported in *The Daily Telegraph*, they were breaking the coronavirus lockdown rules of that time. One of the men, a forty-seven-year-old from Leicester, suffered chest pains during the night and dialled emergency services.

The Mountain Rescue Team was on their way to them when Chris Lewis plunged 500 feet down a ravine. He suffered multiple facial fractures in the fall, including extremely serious damage to his back, spine and neck. Apparently, being left in a wheelchair for the rest of his life 'would be a good outcome'.[7]

Despite the fury aimed at the two campers online, Martin Cotterell from the mountain rescue team said volunteers 'are not there to judge'. *The Daily Telegraph* reported that he said: 'We are there to help. We all love the fells, we are all mountaineers, we go out there because we think we can help people in difficulty. Trying to judge is wrong.'[7]

At the time of the newspaper report on the tragedy, Chris Lewis was still in intensive care. The campers were each fined £200 for breaching coronavirus lockdown laws.

Apparently the first thing Mr Lewis said when he arrived at the hospital was 'How's the other casualty?'

This tragedy might never have happened if the two campers' 'place of safety', as their way of coping during this extraordinary time, was not as hazardous or dysfunctional as a tent high up in the Lake District.

This didn't really have to happen. They shouldn't have been there in the first place. But they felt a need to, which was perhaps their way of dealing with their pandemic panic. Their attempt to escape from stress has now created a lifelong nightmare for someone else.

This catastrophe was not directly caused by the virus. No one here caught it. Instead, the tragedy evolved from a series of actions which were a personal reaction to coping with COVID-19.

This is the true story of the pandemic which will not come to be written for many years: that in the end more suffering might have been caused by the government's and the public's reaction to the pandemic than the virus itself. We need to cope better because it's the catastrophic coping that can kill, perhaps even more so than the contagion itself.

We can act decisively to stop the spread of profound negative reaction; we have done it before. We just seem to have forgotten how – just as we forgot there was an influenza pandemic back at almost exactly the same point in the twentieth century.

At noon on 15 August 1945, Japanese Emperor Hirohito ordered his faithful subjects to stop fighting the war and lay down their arms.[8] Western observers were convinced that as loss of face plays such a central role in Japanese culture, mass suicide might become the culturally admirable escape from disgrace.[9] Japanese citizens might struggle to understand how someone they regarded as a living deity could admit defeat.

How does anyone respond to the humiliation of surrender after the devastation of two nuclear bombs on top of the catastrophe wreaked by the rest of the war? How does one recover psychologically from such a low point?

But Japan has been rebuilt, and the dawn of reconstruction has been dated to a very precise moment: Emperor Hirohito's radio address, which lasted just four minutes.

If you read between the lines, the Emperor's speech was also a spiritual antidote to suicide. Winston Churchill gets all the accolades as the speech maker of the era, but maybe, when all is said and done, it's how the losers live on which has more to teach us.

Might it be that the Emperor of Japan delivered the most consequential words of the twentieth century?

Surrender was officially forbidden in the Japanese military, and Japanese civilians were also expected to choose death in order to protect national pride. 'The hundred million', the propaganda term for the civilians guarding the homeland, might have had to embrace a demise that would be stunning in its immensity,[9] 'like shattered jewels'.

Instead, the Emperor did something completely unexpected.

Emperor Hirohito invoked a generational sense of destiny, and a personal redefining of what is intolerable. Are these sentiments as expressed by the Emperor in his speech the most effective mass suicide prevention intervention in history? Did these words save more Japanese lives from self-destruction and despair than were lost in the whole war?

Just after 11 p.m. on 14 August, the Emperor and his staff confirmed the transcript. The Japanese people were told they were surrendering, but doing so with dignity. It was a massive gamble. The speech was then recorded on a phonograph disc.[10]

Hundreds of army officers stationed around Tokyo heard of the planned radio broadcast, but they considered surrender ignominious. They attacked the Imperial Palace to intercept and destroy the recording. But the attempted coup d'état proved futile, and its leaders were left to commit suicide.[10]

In what became known as the 'Jewel Voice Broadcast', Hirohito's address went out at noon on 15 August. The scratchy recording and the fact that he declaimed in classical Japanese meant at first these words generated considerable misunderstanding.

The Mental Vaccine for COVID-19 may well experience the same reception. This is a radically different approach to anything which has come before. Just as most had never heard their emperor's voice before, many will find these messages difficult to hear.

But within nineteen years, a rebuilt Tokyo was hosting the 1964 Summer Olympic Games; they were opened by the very same Emperor Hirohito.

Yet whether the Olympics should take place at all now in 2021 is dogged by controversy over contagion. If this pandemic has a lesson it is surely this: we neglect the emotional need we all have for concrete positive emblems of survival at our peril.

The next Olympics in Tokyo, where the planet unites for the first time after the pandemic, are more than just games. They are a vital symbol of psychological resilience and rebuilding in a post-pandemic world.

In the future, we are sure to continue to need more of these flags, more moments, more triumphs to inspire and nourish us.

Did Emperor Hirohito's speech at noon on 15 August 1945 contain one of the ingredients, part of the 'secret sauce', in the Mental Vaccine for COVID-19? You decide.

It is according to the dictates of time and fate that we have resolved to pave the way for a grand peace for all the generations to come by enduring the unendurable and suffering what is insufferable ... Cultivate the ways of rectitude, foster nobility of spirit, and work with resolution.

ACKNOWLEDGEMENTS

I should like to thank various collaborators who have helped with this book. These include Professor Adrian Furnham, who introduced me to psychology when I was a student at University College London, and others, who you can find in the references section. The editorial input and advice of Susan Lumsden, Gwyneth Williams and Gary McConnell were most appreciated. Juliet Wilberforce performed heroically in editing the final manuscript. Steven Tucker, Nick Hayward and Nikki Embery of Amberley Publishing did an amazing job in bringing the book to publication so soon.

I hope to publish another analysis soon, focussed on obtaining psychological help from the health service, once psychiatric services have decided to cease self-isolating.

ABOUT THE AUTHOR

Dr Raj Persaud is a Consultant Psychiatrist who has worked as a Consultant at the Bethlem Royal and Maudsley NHS Hospitals in London from 1994 to 2008, and as an Honorary Senior Lecturer at the Institute of Psychiatry, University of London. These are the premier research and training institutions for psychiatry in Europe.

He was also Research Fellow at Johns Hopkins Hospital in the USA and Institute of Neurology at Queens Square. His training in psychiatry since leaving UCH medical school in1986 was entirely at the Institute of Psychiatry and the Bethlem Royal and Maudsley Hospitals. Unusually for a psychiatrist, he also holds a degree in psychology, obtained with First Class Honours, and eight other degrees and diplomas including a Masters in Statistics. He was awarded the Royal College of Psychiatrists' Research Prize and Medal as well as the Maudsley Hospital's own Denis Hill Prize, and the Osler Medal. The Royal College of Psychiatrists also awarded him the Morris Markowe Prize.

In 2004 he was appointed Visiting Professor for Public Understanding of Psychiatry at Gresham College, and he was asked by the Royal College of Psychiatrists to edit its first book aimed at educating the public on psychology and psychiatry. *The Mind: A User's Guide* was published in 2007 and reached the top ten bestseller list. All of his five previous books have been top ten bestsellers. He has contributed a chapter to the Royal College's latest book, *The Female Mind: A User's Guide*.

He has contributed to several established textbooks, including the *Oxford Companion to the Mind* and a chapter in the latest comprehensive textbook of psychiatry for trainees, *Psychiatry – An Evidence Based Text*. He has approaching 100 publications in journals such as the *British Journal of Psychiatry*, the *British Medical Journal* and *The Lancet*.

He was elected Fellow of University College London and the Royal College of Psychiatrists. He has been a supporter of numerous mental health charities including OCD-UK, the Manic Depression Fellowship, Association of Post-Natal Illness, Childline, Action Aid and the Samaritans.

Raj Persaud has delivered many of the annual lectures in British Medicine including the prestigious 2002 Florence Nightingale Lecture, the Whittington Oration, the Annual Oration of the Medical Society of London, and the keynote lecture of the annual conference for National Institute of Clinical Excellence. He gave the widely publicised lecture celebrating the fiftieth anniversary of the foundation of the Samaritans. He has chaired prestigious panels, including the one to choose the International Aventis Science Book Prize for 2002 – the top book prize for science books given annually. He has judged the annual UK Broadcast Medical Journalism Awards, as well as the Health Service Journal Awards, which include the Minister of Health's Award.

The Independent on Sunday conducted a poll among members of the Royal College of Psychiatrists and the Institute of Psychiatry to discover who were the top ten psychiatrists in the UK as rated by fellow psychiatrists. Dr Raj Persaud was the youngest doctor to make it into this esteemed list. *The Times* also placed him as one of the Top Twenty Mental Health Gurus in the world.

His Ted talk has had over 3.5 million views. His *Psychology Today* blog has had over 1.3 million views. His podcasts have had over 30,000 downloads.

NOTES

To the Reader
1. www.samaritans.org email jo@samaritans.org phone 116 123

Preface: Why a Mental Vaccine?
1. Harry and Meghan try interviews without the interviewing – Archewell Audio podcast review Hannah Verdier Tue 29 Dec 2020 17.59 GMT The Guardian https://www.theguardian.com/tv-and-radio/2020/dec/29/archewell-audio-podcast-review-harry-and-meghan-try-interviews-without-the-interviewing
    Archewell Audio podcast review — 'Like Goop but without the fun' James Marriott's verdict on Harry and Meghan's new podcast James Marriott Wednesday December 30 2020, 12.01am, The Times https://www.thetimes.co.uk/article/archewell-audio-podcast-review-like-goop-but-without-the-fun-xg989poht
    'Off to a rocky start': Meghan and Harry's much-hyped Archewell Audio podcast is a right royal miss. By Ed Power 29 December 2020 6:16pm The Daily Telegraph https://www.telegraph.co.uk/radio/what-to-listen-to/rocky-start-meghan-harrys-much-hyped-archewell-audio-podcast/
2. Coronavirus: Dr Radha's five mental health tips for lockdown Dr Radha Modgil from BBC Radio 1's Life Hacks shares her top five tips on how to stay mentally and emotionally well during the coronavirus lockdown, all beginning with the letter C https://www.bbc.co.uk/news/av/newsbeat-52411394
3. How Holmes filled his attic in Baker Street. Paul Jones Radcliffe-on-Trent, Nottinghamshire The Daily Telegraph https://www.telegraph.co.uk/opinion/2021/01/02/letters-guarantee-enough-pfizer-vaccine-will-left-give-recipients/
    Holmes's empty head Rob White London N3 The Daily Telegraph https://www.telegraph.co.uk/opinion/2020/12/31/letters-oxford-vaccine-cause-celebration-time-get-move/
4. Changes to information in working memory depend on distinct removal operations Hyojeong Kim, Harry R. Smolker, Louisa L. Smith, Marie T. Banich & Jarrod A. Lewis-Peacock. Nature Communications | (2020) 11:6239 https://doi.org/10.1038/s41467-020-20085-4 www.nature.com/naturecommunications
5. News Release 17-DEC-2020 How can you declutter your mind? New study offers clues Brain imaging offers insight on how we purge thoughts to

make room for new ones. University of Colorado at Boulder https://www.eurekalert.org/pub_releases/2020-12/uoca-hcy121720.php

Introduction: A Plague of the Absurd

1. Coronavirus: Top NYC doctor takes her own life (https://www.bbc.co.uk/news/world-us-canada-52451094?intlink_from_url=htt …).
2. Top E.R. Doctor Who Treated Virus Patients Dies by Suicide https://www.nytimes.com/2020/04/27/nyregion/new-york-city-doctor-suicide-coronavirus.html
3. British Medical Journal Rapid Response by Dr Raj Persaud https://www.bmj.com/content/369/bmj.m1506/rr
4. BMJ doi: 10.1136/bmj.39317.641146.4E https://www.bmj.com/content/335/7619/567.2 (The Plague, Minerva, BMJ 23 April 2020, BMJ 2020;369:m1506)
5. COVID stress syndrome: Concept, structure, and correlates Steven Taylor Caeleigh A. Landry Michelle M. Paluszek Thomas A. Fergus Dean McKay Gordon J. G. Asmundson Depression and Anxiety 2020 Aug;37(8): 706-714 First published: 05 July 2020 https://doi.org/10.1002/da.23071 V
6. Prevalence of mental disorders and mental health service use in Japan Daisuke Nishi MD, PhD, Hanako Ishikawa MD, PhD, Norito Kawakami MD, PhD First published: 29 May 2019 https://doi.org/10.1111/pcn.12894 Psychiatry and Clinical Neurosciences Volume73, Issue8 August 2019 Pages 458-465
7. Japan suicide rates soar as economy suffers from coronavirus pandemic. Women appear to have been hardest hit even as national figures remain relatively low The Daily Telegraph By Danielle Demetriou Tokyo 11 November 2020 • 10:07am www.telegraph.co.uk/news/2020/11/11/japan-suicide-rates-soar-economy-suffers-coronavirus-pandemic/
   Pandemic raises Japan suicide rate after decade of decline https://www.japantimes.co.jp/news/2021/01/22/national/japan-suicide-rate/
8. Deepening despair Suicide is on the rise among South Korean women The young are especially likely to kill themselves https://www.economist.com/asia/2020/12/12/suicide-is-on-the-rise-among-south-korean-women
9. Exclusive: Number of people seeking help for suicidal thoughts has tripled since lockdown Mental health services said to be 'overflowing' with patients as investigation reveals increases in ambulance call-outs By Laura Donnelly, HEALTH EDITOR and Tony Diver 8 November 2020 • 9:30pm The Daily Telegraph Newspaper https://www.telegraph.co.uk/news/2020/11/08/exclusive-number-people-seeking-help-suicidal-thoughts-has-tripled/
10. Rose, Jacqueline. "Pointing the Finger." London Review of Books 42.9 (2020): n.p. Lrb.co.uk. Web. 2 Jun. 2020.
11. The Plague By Albert Camus May 07, 1991 | ISBN 9780679720218 Penguin Random House.
    ┌ Camus A. La Peste (French), Paris: Gallimard, 1947. The Plague. Translated in English by Stuart Gilbert, London: Hamish Hamilton; 1948.
12. Crime in England and Wales: year ending June 2020 Office of National Statistics https://www.ons.gov.uk/peoplepopulationandcommunity/crimeandjustice/bulletins/crimeinenglandandwales/yearendingjune2020#fraud
13. Go-between paid £21m in taxpayer funds for NHS PPE By Phil Kemp BBC News https://www.bbc.co.uk/news/uk-54974373

14. US jeweller 'was paid £200m by UK to secure PPE' Government faces legal challenge in British courts over contracts but insists 'proper due diligence' was followed By Tony Diver 17 November 2020 • 9:38pm www.telegraph.co.uk/news/2020/11/17/court-papers-us-say-200m-taxpayers-money-paid-firm-had-no-ppe/

15. Millions wasted by government on useless PPE could have paid for free school meals, Labour says Government spent £150m on masks that cannot be used Jon Stone Policy Correspondent @joncstone Monday 26 October 2020 22:29 https://www.independent.co.uk/news/uk/politics/free-school-meals marcus-rashford-labour-boris-johnson-tories-ppe-cost-b1350425.html

16. Ministers reliant on companies owned by the Chinese state By Ben Gartside At least £2.5bn of the UK's PPE supply was made in Chinese factories, according to Telegraph analysis. The Daily Telegraph https://www.telegraph.co.uk/business/2020/12/22/consultants-airlines-china-cashed-scramble-ppe/

17. How consultants, airlines and China cashed in on PPE scramble At least £175m of taxpayer money has been spent on consultants – but the true cost is likely to be much higher By Michael O'Dwyer and Ben Gartside 22 December 2020 • 3:00pm The Daily Telegraph https://www.telegraph.co.uk/business/2020/12/22/consultants-airlines-china-cashed-scramble-ppe/

18. German hospitals accused of exploiting coronavirus to secure funds. Hospitals kept ICU beds empty because it was 'more lucrative' than treating patients, says MP By Justin Huggler BERLIN 3 December 2020 5:32pm The Daily Telegraph https://www.telegraph.co.uk/news/2020/12/03/german-hospitals-accused-exploiting-coronavirus-secure-funds/

19. Hand sanitiser gels sold online fail Which? tests Three of the 18 hand sanitisers tested didn't contain enough alcohol to effectively kill the COVID-19 virus or other germs. Read more: https://www.which.co.uk/news/2020/12/hand-sanitisers-sold-online-fail-which-tests/ – Which?

20. Police appeal for information over fake 'nude game show' footage Two men reported being invited to a hotel to take part in nude "challenges" for footage By Nisha Mal 10:49, 12 DEC 2020 www.grimsbytelegraph.co.uk/news/uk-world-news/police-appeal-information-over-fake-4792540

21. East Anglian Bonnie and Clyde 'leave trail of unpaid pub bills' Couple accused of charming their way out of paying for food, drink and accommodation Archie Bland Tue 17 Nov 2020 17.12 GMT Last modified on Tue 17 Nov 2020 18.29 GMT The Guardian https://www.theguardian.com/uk-news/2020/nov/17/east-anglian-bonnie-and-clyde-leave-trail-of-unpaid-pub-bills

    Police hunt for 'dine and dash' couple who swindled up to a DOZEN pubs and restaurants by fleeing without paying for meals and hotel stays during ten-month crime spree By James Gant for Mailonline www.dailymail.co.uk/news/article-8953273/Norfolk-Suffolk-Police-hunt-dine-dash-couple-swindled-DOZEN-hospitality-venues.html 10:52, 16 November 2020

22. The Journal of Social Encounters Volume 4 Issue 2 Article 10 2020 Rereading Albert Camus' The Plague During a Pandemic: Of Plagues and Nazis: Camus' Journey from Moral Nihilism Stephen I. Wagner College of St. Benedict/St. John's University

23. Married actors become Hermes drivers as theatres shut down. Leading lady and her actor husband were forced to find work after the pandemic shuttered London theatres By Anita Singh, Arts and Entertainment Editor 17 October 2020 • 3:00pm www.telegraph.co.uk/news/2020/10/17/married-actors-become-hermes-drivers-theatres-shut-deliver-parcel/

24. After Dr. Lorna Breen Died By Suicide in April, Her Family Took Up a Cause They Never Wanted By Jordan Grantham September 10, 2020 www.acepnow.com/article/after-dr-lorna-breen-died-by-suicide-in-april-her-family-took-up-a-cause-they-never-wanted/3/

25. Gratitude 19 Nov. 2015 Oliver Sacks

26. The Meditations By Marcus Aurelius Written 167 A.C.E. Translated by George Long

27. Hankey M. Memorandum to Committee of Imperial Defence, July 2, 1924 (The National Archives of the UK, CAB46/3 ARP/8).

28. Basu D. The Plague by Albert Camus, the COVID-19 Pandemic, and the Role of Social Psychiatry – Lessons Shared, Lessons Learned. World Soc Psychiatry 2020;2:51-6

1 Why Worry Is More Contagious than Any Virus

1. Jos Brosschot, Bart Verkuil and Julian Thayer The default response to uncertainty and the importance of perceived safety in anxiety and stress: An evolution-theoretical perspective Journal of Anxiety Disorders Volume 41, June 2016, Pages 22-34

2. Vigilance Behaviour in Grazing African Antelopes In: Behaviour Author: R. Underwood 1 Online Publication Date: 01 Jan 1982 In: Volume 79: Issue 2-4 81–107

3. How to escape from a lion or cheetah — the science By Helen Briggs BBC News Published 24 January 2018 www.bbc.co.uk/news/science-environment-42792190

4. Why Zebras Don't Get Ulcers: A Guide To Stress, Stress Related Disease And Coping, R. M. Sapolsky, W. H. Freeman & Co., New York, 1993. No. of pages: 368,

5. Coronavirus could travel five metres through air, study finds Scientists isolate infectious particles of the virus at a distance of up to 4.8 metres from patients being treated in hospital By Phoebe Southworth15 August 2020 • 5:00pm The Daily Telegraph https://www.telegraph.co.uk/news/2020/08/15/coronavirus-could-travel-five-metres-air-study-finds/

6. Aerosol and surface stability of HCoV-19 (SARS-CoV-2) compared to SARS-CoV-1 Neeltje vanDoremalen, Trenton Bushmaker, Dylan Morris, Myndi Holbrook, Amandine Gamble, Brandi Williamson, Azaibi Tamin, Jennifer Harcourt, Natalie Thornburg, Susan Gerber, Jamie Lloyd-Smith, Emmie de Wit, Vincent Munster doi: https://doi.org/10.1101/2020.03.09.20033217 Now published in The New England Journal of Medicine doi: 10.1056/NEJMc2004973

7. Evidence of Long-Distance Droplet Transmission of SARS-CoV-2 by Direct Air Flow in a Restaurant in Korea Keun-Sang Kwon, Jung-Im Park, Young Joon Park, Don-Myung Jung, Ki-Wahn Ryu, and Ju-Hyung Lee, J Korean Med Sci. 2020 Nov 30;35(46):e415. English. Published online Nov 23, 2020.

https://doi.org/10.3346/jkms.2020.35.e415 2020 The Korean Academy of Medical Sciences.

8. First death from COVID-19 reinfection reported in the Netherlands By Georgina Hayes 13 October 2020 • 1:37pm The Daily Telegraph Newspaper https://www.telegraph.co.uk/global-health/science-and-disease/first-death-covid-19-reinfection-reported-netherlands/

9. The Motivated Mind R Persaud Random House – 2006

10. Goyal M, Singh S, Sibinga EMS, et al. Meditation Programs for Psychological Stress and Well-being: A Systematic Review and Meta-analysis. JAMA Intern Med. 2014;174(3):357–368. doi:10.1001/jamainternmed.2013.13018

11. Mindfulness meditation: Do-it-yourself medicalization of every moment Kristin K. Barker Social Science & Medicine Volume 106, April 2014, Pages 168-176

12. Why Meditate When You Could Just Rest? Raj Persaud Arch Intern Med. 2006;166(22):2553-2554. doi:10.1001/archinte.166.22.2553-b

13. Marr AJ Relaxation and muscular tension: a biobehavioristic explanation. Int J Stress Manage 2006;13131- 153

14. Roy F. Baumeister, Kathleen D. Vohs, Jennifer L. Aaker & Emily N. Garbinsky (2013) Some key differences between a happy life and a meaningful life, The Journal of Positive Psychology, 8:6, 505-516, DOI: 10.1080/17439760.2013.830764

15. Covid: 'Pressure' led to Wrexham care home owner's suicide. https://www.bbc.co.uk/news/uk-wales-55087446

16. Sperry TS, Thompson CK, Wingfield JC. Effects of acute treatment with 8-OH-DPAT and fluoxetine on aggressive behaviour in male song sparrows (Melospiza melodia morphna). J Neuroendocrinol. 2003 Feb;15(2):150-60. doi: 10.1046/j.1365-2826.2003.00968.x. PMID: 12535157.

17. Heidi A.N Perreault, Katharine Semsar, John Godwin, Fluoxetine treatment decreases territorial aggression in a coral reef fish, Physiology & Behavior, Volume 79, Issues 4–5, 2003, Pages 719-724,ISSN 0031-9384, https://doi.org/10.1016/S0031-9384(03)00211-7 (http://www.sciencedirect.com/science/article/pii/S0031938403002117)

18. A Surprising Approach for Coping With COVID-19 Stress. Has psychology been thinking about stress in the wrong way up until now? https://www.psychologytoday.com/gb/blog/slightly-blighty/202010/surprising-approach-coping-covid-19-stress

2 How to Panic Properly over the Pandemic

1. Anthony R. Mawson (2005). Understanding Mass Panic and Other Collective Responses to Threat and Disaster. Psychiatry: Interpersonal and Biological Processes: Vol. 68, No. 2, pp. 95-113. https://doi.org/10.1521/psyc.2005.68.2.95

2. Internet Searches for Acute Anxiety During the Early Stages of the COVID-19 Pandemic. John Ayers, Eric Leas, Derek Johnson, Adam Poliak, Benjamin Althouse, Mark Dredze, Alicia Nobles. JAMA Intern Med. Published online August 24, 2020. doi:10.1001/jamainternmed.2020.3305

3. People living alone 'twice as likely to test positive for COVID-19' ONS data shows those in one-person households more likely to test positive on a swab test

than those in two-person set-ups. Gabriella Swerling, Social and Religious affairs Editor 18 August 2020 • 4:18pm. www.telegraph.co.uk/news/2020/08/18/people-living-alone-twice-likely-test-positive-covid-19-reveal/

4. The psychology of protecting the UK public against external threat: COVID-19 and the Blitz compared Historical Review Volume 7, Issue 11, P991-996, November 01, 2020 Prof Edgar Jones, PhD The Lancet Psychiatry Published: August 27, 2020 DOI:https://doi.org/10.1016/S2215-0366(20)30342-4

5. "Sully" Sullenberger and the Miracle on the Hudson: A Lesson in Heroism for Oral and Maxillofacial Surgeons Leon A. Assael, Journal of Oral and Maxillofacial Surgery Volume 67, Issue 4, P711-712, APRIL 01, 2009

6. January 27, 2015 What I Learned About Adverse Events From Captain Sully It's Not What You Think Marjorie Podraza Stiegler, MD JAMA. 2015;313(4):361-362. doi:10.1001/jama.2014.16025

7. Applying aviation factors to oral and maxillofacial surgery – the human element W. Smith Anish Patel Howard Brunt Peter A. Brennan British Journal of Oral and Maxillofacial Surgery Volume 51, Issue 1, January 2013, Pages 8-13

8. Does 'Sully' Reveal How To Cope With Anxiety? Does the Hollywood version of heroism hide the truth about coping with fear? https://www.psychologytoday.com/us/blog/slightly-blighty/201703/does-sully-reveal-how-cope-anxiety?amp

9. How People Panicked Over the Pandemic https://www.psychologytoday.com/gb/blog/slightly-blighty/202009/how-people-panicked-over-the-pandemic

10. Encyclopedia of Mental Health 2nd Edition Editor in Chief: Howard Friedman
ISBN: 9780123970459 Imprint: Academic Press Published Date: 17th September 2015

3 Living with Loss during Lockdown

1. Grenfell firefighter comforted trapped woman with toddler by saying she would be saved when he knew she would not, inquiry hears Zainab Deen watched her child succumb to the smoke before she begged to die herself Harriet Agerholm@HarrietAgerholm Thursday 02 August 2018 19:11 https://www.independent.co.uk/news/uk/home-news/grenfell-tower-fire-firefighter-lied-saving-residents-zainab-deen-jeremiah-a8474951.html

2. Powell, Steve; Butollo, Willi; Hagl, Maria. 'Missing or killed: The differential effect on mental health in women in Bosnia and Herzegovina of the confirmed or unconfirmed loss of their husbands'. European Psychologist, Vol 15(3), 2010, 185-192

3. Carina Heeke, Nadine Stammel and Christine Knaevelsrud. 'When hope and grief intersect: Rates and risks of prolonged grief disorder among bereaved individuals and relatives of disappeared persons in Colombia'. Journal of Affective Disorders 173 (2015) 59–64

4. Sir Patrick Stewart: 'At 80, I'm still in therapy to deal with seeing my mother beaten by my father' The veteran actor took decades to speak about the domestic abuse he witnessed as a child. He tells Guy Kelly how it still afflicts him today. By Guy Kelly 5 December 2020

6:00am. The Daily Telegraph www.telegraph.co.uk/men/the-filter/sir-patrick-stewartat-80-still-therapy-deal-seeing-mother-beaten/

5. Grief counselling a waste of time, say psychologists By Raj Persaud 04 June 2005 • 00:01 am www.telegraph.co.uk/news/uknews/1491354/Grief-counselling-a-waste-of-time-say-psychologists.html

Stroebe, M., Stroebe, W., Schut, H., Zech, E., & van den Bout, J. (2002). Does disclosure of emotions facilitate recovery from bereavement? Evidence from two prospective studies. Journal of Consulting and Clinical Psychology, 70(1), 169–178. https://doi.org/10.1037/0022-006X.70.1.169

6. Prince Harry reveals he's been in therapy for seven years to cope with the death of his mother Harry and Meghan spoke at their first event since stepping down as Royals. by Emily Gulla Feb 8, 2020

https://www.cosmopolitan.com/uk/reports/a30821572/prince-harry-therapy-seven-years/#:~:text=Prince per cent20Harry per cent20and per cent20Meghan per cent20Markle, per cent2C per cent20Princess per cent20Diana per cent2C per cent20in per cent201997.

7. Parental death during childhood and depression in young adults — a national cohort study. Berg L, Rostila M, Hjern A. J Child Psychol Psychiatry. 2016 Sep;57(9):1092-8.

8. Gratitude, psychological well-being, and perceptions of posttraumatic growth in adults who lost a parent in childhood. Greene N, McGovern K. Death Studies. 2017 Feb 17:1-11.

9. Coping With Not Knowing What Happened to a Missing Loved One https://www.psychologytoday.com/gb/blog/slightly-blighty/201706/coping-not-knowing-what-happened-missing-loved-one

10. Does Prince Harry Reveal How To Cope With Loss? https://www.psychologytoday.com/gb/blog/slightly-blighty/201704/does-prince-harry-reveal-how-cope-loss

4 Could the Pandemic Result in 50,000 Suicides Worldwide?

1. Blaustein M, Fleming A: Suicide from the Golden Gate Bridge. Am J Psychiatry 2009; 1111–1116

2. Suicide Prevention on the Golden Gate Bridge Jacobs John, M.D. 1 April 2010 American Journal of Psychiatry, Vol. 167, No. 4

Drs. Blaustein and Fleming Reply Mel Blaustein, M.D., and Anne Fleming, M.D., M.S. 1 April 2010 | American Journal of Psychiatry, Vol. 167, No. 4

3. Preliminary Investigation of the Association Between COVID-19 and Suicidal Thoughts and Behaviors in the U.S. Brooke Ammerman, Taylor Burke, Ross Jacobucci, Kenneth McClure. Preprint DOI 10.31234/osf.io/68djp PsyArXiv Preprints

4. Economic suicides in the Great Recession in Europe and North America Aaron Reeves, Martin McKee and David Stuckler. British Journal of Psychiatry. Volume 205, Issue 3 September 2014, pp. 246-247

5. Increased Risk of Suicide Due to Economic and Social Impacts of Social Distancing Measures to Address the COVID-19 Pandemic: A Forecast. Carl Weems, Victor Carrion, Bethany McCurdy and Mikaela Scozzafava.   https://www.researchgate.net/profile/Carl_Weems/

publication/340487993_Increased_Risk_of_Suicide_Due_to_Economic_
and_Social_Impacts_of_Social_Distancing_Measures_to_Address_the_
COVID-19_Pandemic_A_Forecast/links/5e8c925d4585150839c708de/
Increased-Risk-of-Suicide-Due-to-Economic-and-Social-Impacts-of-Social-
Distancing-Measures-to-Address-the-COVID-19-Pandemic-A-Forecast.
pdfreports

6. Mark D. Griffiths, Mohammed A. Mamun COVID-19 suicidal behavior
among couples and suicide pacts: Case study evidence from press reports
Psychiatry Research Volume 289, July 2020, 113105

7. Seiden RH: Where are they now? a follow-up study of suicide attempters
from the Golden Gate Bridge. Suicide Life Threat Behav 1978; 8:203–216

8. November of the Soul: The Enigma of Suicide By George Howe Colt Simon
and Shuster 2006

9. Study: Some May Seek to Die by Suicide from COVID-19 https://
www.psychologytoday.com/gb/blog/slightly-blighty/202004/
study-some-may-seek-die-suicide-covid-19

5 Don't Cry for Me, Corona

1. Picó, A., Gračanin, A., Gadea, M. et al. How Visible Tears Affect Observers'
Judgements and Behavioral Intentions: Sincerity, Remorse, and Punishment.
J Nonverbal Behav 44, 215–232 (2020). https://doi.org/10.1007/
s10919-019-00328-9

2. Covid: Doctor 'has shed more tears than ever' Published 28 December 2020
https://www.bbc.co.uk/news/uk-wales-55460248

3. Why is Radio 3 downgrading classical music to a trendy form of therapy?
Ivan Hewett 21 February 2021 • 6:00am The Daily Telegraph https://
www.telegraph.co.uk/radio/what-to-listen-to/radio-3-downgrading-
classical-music-trendy-form-therapy/

4. Gracanin, A., Bylsma, L. M., & Vingerhoets, A. J. J. M. (2018). Why
only humans shed emotional tears: Evolutionary and cultural perspectives.
Human Nature, 29(2), 104–133.

5. Vingerhoets, A. J. J. M. (2013). Why only humans weep: Unravelling the
mysteries of tears. Oxford: Oxford University Press

6. Lauren M. Bylsma, Ad J. J. M. Vingerhoets, and Jonathan Rottenberg
(2008). When is Crying Cathartic? An International Study. Journal of
Social and Clinical Psychology: Vol. 27, No. 10, pp. 1165-1187. https://doi.
org/10.1521/jscp.2008.27.10.1165

7. Lauren M. Bylsma, Marcel A. Croon, Ad.J.J.M. Vingerhoets, Jonathan
Rottenberg, When and for whom does crying improve mood? A daily diary
study of 1004 crying episodes, Journal of Research in Personality, Volume
45, Issue 4, 2011, Pages 385-392.

8. Elsbach, K. D., & Bechky, B. A. (2017). How observers assess crying in
professional work contexts. Academy of Management Discoveries. https://
doi.org/10.5465/amd.2016.0025.

9. Gamliel, T. (2010). "She who mourns will cry": Emotion and expertise in
Yemeni-Israeli wailing. Journal of Anthropological Research, 66, 485–503

10. Harbsmeier, M. (1987). Why do the Indians cry? Culture and History, 1,
90–114.

Why Do the Indians Cry?Author(s): Michael Harbsmeier Source: Etnofoor, 1988, Jaarg. 1, Nr. 1 (1988), pp. 57-77

11. Men Don't Cry, Women Do: Transcending Gender Stereotypes of Grief (Series in Death, Dying, and Bereavement) Paperback – 20 Jan. 2000 by Kenneth J. Doka (Author), Terry L. Martin (Author)

12. Culture and Crying: Prevalences and Gender Differences Dianne A. van Hemert, Fons J. R. van de Vijver, Ad J. J. M. Vingerhoets Cross-Cultural Research Vol 45, Issue 4, 2011

13. Jaeschke, A. & Sachs, M. (2012). 100,000 miles closer to a definition of mental toughness: The farther you run, the more the mind dominates. Marathon & Beyond, 16(5), 44-67.

6 How COVID Killed Comedy: Does Humour Really Help Heal?

1. At Witz End: Theory in a Time of Plague Elizabeth Rottenberg Derrida Today 2020 Volume 13, Issue 2 / 210–216

2. 49 Coronavirus and Quarantine Jokes to Retrain Your Face to Smile It's a pundemic. By Emily Kelleher Updated Nov 19 2020, 11:57 AM https://www.fatherly.com/play/best-coronavirus-jokes/

3. Psychotic traits in comedians Published online by Cambridge University Press: 02 January 2018 Victoria Ando Gordon Claridge and Ken Clark The British Journal of Psychiatry, Volume 204, Issue 5, May 2014, pp. 341 – 345 DOI: https://doi.org/10.1192/bjp.bp.113.134569

4. The moderating effect of humor style on the relationship between interpersonal predictors of suicide and suicidal ideation Raymond P.Tucker La Rick R. Wingate Victoria M. O'Keefe Meredith L. Slish Matt R Judah Sarah Rhoades-Kerswill Personality and Individual Differences Volume 54, Issue 5, April 2013, Pages 610-615

5. Does comedy kill? A retrospective, longitudinal cohort, nested case–control study of humour and longevity in 53 British comedians Simon Stewart David R.Thompson International Journal of Cardiology Volume 180, 1 February 2015, Pages 258-261

6. The Big Five personality traits of professional comedians compared to amateur comedians, comedy writers, and college students Gil Greengross Geoffrey F.Miller Personality and Individual Differences Volume 47, Issue 2, July 2009, Pages 79-83

7. Gallows Humor in Medicine Author(s): Katie Watson The Hastings Center Report, Vol. 41, No. 5 (September-October 2011), pp. 37-45 Published by: The Hastings Center Stable URL: https://www.jstor.org/stable/4124130

8. Crosby, Alfred W. (1989), America's Forgotten Pandemic: The Influenza of 1918, Cambridge, New York: Cambridge University Press.

7 Does COVID Also Kill by Boring You to Death?

1. Vatican demands an explanation from Instagram after Pope Francis's account liked a photo of a Brazilian model dressed as a schoolgirl. www.dailymail.co.uk/news/article-8969923/Vatican-demands-answers-Instagram-Popes-model-photo-like.html

2. The Boredom Pandemic https://www.project-syndicate.org/commentary/ covid19-lockdown-causes-dangerous-boredom-by-raj-persaud-2020- 04?barrier=accesspaylog

3. Today you're bored, tomorrow you're ill. https://www.independent. co.uk/life-style/health-and-families/health-news/health-today-youre- bored-tomorrow-youre-ill-raj-persaud-explains-a-phenomenon-that-can- cause-air-1500829.html Raj Persaud Tuesday 30 March 1993 00:02

4. Bloom AJ, Yorges SL, Ruhl, AJ. Enhancing student motivation: Extensions from job enrichment theory and practice. Teaching Psychol 2000;27:135–7.

5. Licata JW, Mowen JC, Harris EG, Brown TJ. On the trait antecedents and outcomes of service worker job resourcefulness: a hierarchical model approach. J Acad Marketing Sci2003;31:256–71.

6. Boredom at Work: A Neglected Concept Cynthia D. Fisherl Human RelationsVolume: 46 issue: 3, page(s): 395-417 Issue published: March 1, 1993

7. Rothbard NP. Enriching or depleting? The dynamics of engagement in work and family roles. Admin Sci Q2001;46:655–84.

8. Niehoff BP, Moorman RH, Blakely G, Fuller J. The influence of empowerment and job enrichment on employee loyalty in a downsizing environment. Group & Organization Management 2001;26:93–113.

9. "It's Going to be Extra Fun!": Analysis of an Atypical Case of Teen Homicide as Leisure Behavior D J Williams and Jolene Vincent Volume63, Issue6 November 2018 Pages 1914-1916

10. Van Tilburg, W. A. P., & Igou, E. R. (2016). Going to political extremes in response to boredom. European Journal of Social Psychology, 46(6), 687–699. https://doi.org/10.1002/ejsp.2205

11. 'Boredom Is Polarizing: The Effects of Boredom on Ideological Extremes' Wilson, Gillian.The New School, ProQuest Dissertations Publishing, 2019. 13881861.

12. Risk-taking increases under boredom Kılıç, Ayşenur and Van Tilburg, Wijnand AP and Igou, Eric R (2019) Journal of Behavioral Decision Making. ISSN 0894-3257 Volume 33, Issue 3, 1 July 2020, Pages 257-269

13. Moynihan, A. B., Igou, E. R., & van Tilburg, W. A. P. (2017). Boredom increases impulsiveness: A meaning-regulation perspective. Social Psychology, 48(5), 293–309. https://doi.org/10.1027/1864-9335/a000317

14. Psychotherapy with the Boring Patient Graeme J. Taylor, M.B. The Canadian Journal of Psychiatry First Published April 1, 1984 Research Article Find in PubMed https://doi.org/10.1177/070674378402900306 Vol 29, Issue 3, 1984

15. It's unofficial: cricket club knocks world record for six Buckingham News Jenna Outhwaite September 3, 2020 https://buckingham.news/its-unofficial- cricket-club-knocks-world-record-for-six/#:~:text=Buckingham%20 Town%20Cricket%20Club%20attempted,lengths%20of%20a%20 cricket%20pitch.

    Most cricket runs between the wickets in 12 hours (team) https://www. guinnessworldrecords.com/world-records/622546-greatest-distance-run- between-the-wickets-in-12-hours-team

    Cricket club breaks world record for most runs in 12 hours By Patrick Sawer The Daily Telegraph 21 November 2020 5:00pm https://www.telegraph. co.uk/news/2020/11/21/cricket-club-breaks-world-record-runs-12-hours/

16. Luke Rhinehart, whose debut novel remained a lasting influence on pop culture 21st December 2020 Obituary: By Neil Cooper The Herald https://www.heraldscotland.com/opinion/18960191.obituary-luke-rhinehart-whose-debut-novel-remained-lasting-influence-pop-culture/

Three days with The Dice Man: 'I never wrote for money or fame' Tanya Gold Sat 4 Mar 2017 13.07 GMT The Guardian https://www.theguardian.com/books/2017/mar/04/three-days-dice-man-never-wrote-money-fame-tanya-gold

Who is the real Dice Man? By Emmanuel Carrère The Guardian Thu 7 Nov 2019 06.00 GMT https://www.theguardian.com/news/2019/nov/07/the-dice-man-elusive-author-luke-rhinehart-george-cockroft-emmanuel-carrere

George Cockcroft, author who as 'Luke Rhinehart' found fame with his book The Dice Man – obituary By Telegraph Obituaries 26 November 2020 • 5:46pmThe Daily Telegraph https://www.telegraph.co.uk/obituaries/2020/11/26/george-cockcroft-author-luke-rhinehart-found-fame-book-dice/

17. Ground Hog Day movie script https://www.imsdb.com/scripts/Groundhog-Day.html

18. How to improve your motivation at work BMJ 2004; 329 doi: https://doi.org/10.1136/sbmj.0410365 (Published 01 October 2004) Cite this as: BMJ 2004;329:0410365 Dr Raj Persaud

8 The People Who Have Spent Twenty Years Preparing for Coronavirus

1. Mota NB, Weissheimer J, Ribeiro M, de Paiva M, Avilla-Souza J, Simabucuru G, et al. (2020) Dreaming during the COVID-19 pandemic: Computational assessment of dream reports reveals mental suffering related to fear of contagion. PLoS ONE 15(11): e0242903. doi:10.1371/journal.pone.0242903

2. Rosenwald, G. C., Mendelsohn, G. A., Fontana, A., & Portz, A. T. (1966). An action test of hypotheses concerning the anal personality. Journal of Abnormal Psychology, 71(4), 304–309. https://doi.org/10.1037/h0023 58

3. Influence of perceived threat of COVID-19 and HEXACO personality traits on toilet paper stockpiling Lisa Garbe, Richard Rau, Theo Toppe https://doi.org/10.1371/journal.pone.0234232 PLOS One

4. OCD: 'I spent 20 years preparing for the coronavirus pandemic'. https://www.bbc.co.uk/news/stories-52564434

5. The other side of COVID-19: Impact on obsessive compulsive disorder (OCD) and hoarding Dr Debanjan Banerjee Psychiatry Res. 2020 Jun; 288: 112966 Published online 2020 Apr 11. doi: 10.1016/j.psychres.2020.112966 PMCID: PMC7151248 PMID: 32334276

6. The aviator on the couch https://www.independent.co.uk/arts-entertainment/films/features/the-aviator-on-the-couch-24442.html

7. Examination of racial differences in assessment of OCD symptoms and obsessive beliefs. Kevin D.Wu Sara V.Wyman Journal of Obsessive-Compulsive and Related Disorders Volume 10, July 2016, Pages 10-18

8. Gender differences in obsessive-compulsive disorder: Findings from a large Indian sample. Anish Cherian, Janardhanan Narayanaswamy, Biju Viswanath, Nishi Guru, Cilna George, Suresh Bada Math, Thennarasu Kandavel and Y.C. Janardhan Reddy Asian Journal of Psychiatry 9 (2014) 17–21

9. Fullana MA, Mataix-Cols D, Caspi A, Harrington H, Grisham JR, Moffitt TE, Poulton R: Obsessions and compulsions in the community: prevalence, interference, help-seeking, developmental stability, and co-occurring psychiatric conditions. Am J Psychiatry 2009; 166:329–336

10. New poll finds ethnic minority groups less likely to want COVID vaccine 16 December 2020 https://www.rsph.org.uk/about-us/news/new-poll-finds-bame-groups-less-likely-to-want-covid-vaccine.html

11. Race and Trust Sandra Susan Smith Annual Review of Sociology 2010 36:1, 453-475

12. Ruscio AM, Stein DJ, Chiu WT, Kessler RC: The epidemiology of obsessivecompulsive disorder in the National Comorbidity Survey Replication. Mol Psychiatry 2008; Aug 26 (Epub ahead of print)

    Salkovskis PM. Cognitive–behavioural approaches to the understanding of obsessive–compulsive problems. In R. M. Rapee (Ed.), Current controversies in the anxiety disorders (pp. 103–133). New York: Guilford Press 1996.

    Salkovskis, P. M., Wroe, A. L., Gledhill, A., Morrison, N., Forrester, E., Richards, C., et al. (2000). Responsibility attitudes and interpretations are characteristic of obsessive compulsive disorder. Behaviour Research and Therapy, 38, 347–372.

    Luciano, J. V., Algarabel, S., Toma´ s, J. M., & Martı´nez, J. L. (2005). Development and validation of the thought control ability questionnaire. Personality and Individual Differences, 38, 997–1008.

    Rheaume J, Freeston MH, Ladouceur R, Bouchard C, Gallant L, Talbot F, Vallieeres A Functional and dysfunctional perfectionists: are they different on compulsive-like behaviors? Behaviour Research and Therapy 38 (2000) 119-128

    Asian community's 'contamination fear' could keep them virus-free https://www.easterneye.biz/asian-communitys-contamination-fearcould-keep-them-virus-free/

    Stein MB: Worrying About Obsessions and Compulsions. Am J Psychiatry 2009 166: 271-273

9 *Is the Pandemic Leading to a New Normal of Revenge Porn?*

1. Revenge Porn and Mental Health: A Qualitative Analysis of the Mental Health Effects of Revenge Porn on Female Survivors. Samantha Bates. Feminist Criminology 1–21 2016 sagepub.com/journals DOI: 10.1177/1557085116654565

2. 'Revenge porn new normal' after cases surge in lockdown. By Cristina Criddle, BBC Technology report-er. https://www.bbc.co.uk/news/technology-54149682

3. Stroud, S. R. (2014). The dark side of the online self: A pragmatist critique of the growing plague of re-venge porn. Journal of Mass Media Ethics: Exploring Questions of Media Morality, 29, 168-183. doi:10.1080/08900523.2014.91797
4. Citron, D. K., & Franks, M. A. (2014). Criminalizing revenge porn. Wake Forest Law Review, 49, 345-391.
5. Wlodarski, R., Dunbar, R.I.M. Examining the Possible Functions of Kissing in Romantic Relationships. Arch Sex Behav 42, 1415–1423 (2013). https://doi.org/10.1007/s10508-013-0190-1
6. Haselton, M. G., & Buss, D. M. (2000). Error management theory: A new perspective on biases in cross-sex mind reading. Journal of Personality and Social Psychology, 78(1), 81–91. https://doi.org/10.1037/0022-3514.78.1.81

10 *Do Psychopaths Secure More Sex despite Social Distancing?*

1. Peter Florjancic obituary Ski-jumping inventor who held more than 400 patents, competed in the Winter Games, duped the Nazis and lived the high life in Monte Carlo Tuesday December 01 2020, 12.01am, The Times https://www.thetimes.co.uk/article/peter-florjancic-obituary-nxj57f59r

   Peter Florjancic: Story of ski-jumping inventor who escaped the Nazis By Gareth Evans BBC News Published 21 November 2020 https://www.bbc.co.uk/news/world-europe-54991711

   Peter Florjančič, inventor behind scores of gadgets including a prototype airbag – obituary He held more than 400 patents and made and lost several fortunes By Telegraph Obituaries 18 November 2020 • 8:48pm The Daily Telegraph https://www.telegraph.co.uk/obituaries/2020/11/18/peter-florjancic-inventor-behind-scores-gadgets-including-prototype/
2. Eunsoo Choi, Taekyun Hur. Is Reading Sexual Intention Truly Functional? The Impact of Perceiving a Partner's Sexual Intention on Courtship Initiation Behaviors, Archives of Sexual Behavior 42, 1525–1533 (2013). https://doi.org/10.1007/s10508-013-0153-6
3. Carolina de Weerth, Akko Kalma. Gender Differences in Awareness of Courtship Initiation Tactics. Sex Roles 32, 717–734 (1995). https://doi.org/10.1007/BF01560186
4. O'Brien DT, Geher G, Gallup AC, Garcia JR, Kaufman SB. Self-Perceived Mating Intelligence Predicts Sexual Behavior in College Students: Empirical Validation of a Theoretical Construct. Imagination, Cognition and Personality. 2010;29(4):341-362. doi:10.2190/IC.29.4.e
5. Hypersexuality in college students: The role of psychopathy Rebecca M. Kastner Martin Sellbom Personality and Individual Differences Volume 53, Issue 5, October 2012, Pages 644-649
6. O'Connell, K., Berluti, K., Rhoads, S. A., & Marsh, A. (2020, June 15). Reduced social distancing during the COVID-19 pandemic is associated with antisocial behaviors in an online United States sample. https://doi.org/10.31234/osf.io/ezypg
7. Kosson, D. S., Kelly, J. C., & White, J. W. (1997). Psychopathy-related traits predict self-reported sexual aggression among college men. Journal of Interpersonal Violence, 12(2), 241–254. https://doi.org/10.1177/088626097012002006

8. Luna C. Muñoz, Roxanne Khan, and Laura Cordwell (2011). Sexually Coercive Tactics Used by University Students: A Clear Role for Primary Psychopathy. Journal of Personality Disorders: Vol. 25, No. 1, pp. 28-40.

9. Why Male and Female Psychopaths Get More Sex Psychological Research Uncovers Character Traits Which Predict Sexual Success www.psychologytoday.com/gb/blog/slightly-blighty/201508/why-male-and-female-psychopaths-get-more-sex

10. Pre-pandemic disgust proneness predicts increased coronavirus anxiety and safety behaviors: Evidence for a diathesis-stress model Rebecca C.Cox Sarah C.Jessup Maxwell J.Luber Bunmi O.Olatunji Journal of Anxiety Disorders Volume 76, December 2020, 102315

11. Effects of Subjective Sexual Arousal on Sexual, Pathogen, and Moral Disgust Sensitivity in Women and Men Ellen M. Lee, James K. Ambler & Brad J. Sagarin Archives of Sexual Behavior volume 43, pages1115–1121(2014)Cite this article

12. Evolution and Human Behavior Volume 36, Issue 3, May 2015, Pages 199-205 Disgust and mating strategy Laith Al-Shawaf David M.G.Lewis David M.Buss

13. Ugh! That's So Disgusting! Repulsion Predicts Your Sex Life https://www.psychologytoday.com/gb/blog/slightly-blighty/201508/ugh-thats-so-disgusting-repulsion-predicts-your-sex-life

11 Loneliness under Lockdown

1. Beyonce admits inauguration miming Published1 February 2013 https://www.bbc.co.uk/news/entertainment-arts-21290682

2. Coronavirus (COVID-19): dealing with awkward social situations – guidance Published: 7 Dec 2020 https://www.gov.scot/publications/coronavirus-covid-19-dealing-with-awkward-social-situations---guidance/

3. Stefanie K. Johnson, Traci Sitzmann, Anh Thuy Nguyen, Don't hate me because I'm beautiful: Acknowledging appearance mitigates the 'beauty is beastly' effect, Organizational Behavior and Human Decision Processes, Volume 125, Issue 2, 2014, Pages 184-192, ISSN 0749-5978, https://doi.org/10.1016/j.obhdp.2014.09.006.

4. Social perception and interpersonal behavior: On the self-fulfilling nature of social stereotypes. Pages 656-666. Snyder, Mark; Tanke, Elizabeth D.; Berscheid, Ellen Journal of Personality and Social Psychology 1977 Volume 35, Issue 9 (Sep)

5. Dorsha Hayes. The Archetypal Nature of Stage Fright. Art Psychotherapy. Volume 2, Issues 3–4, 1975, Pages 279-281
    Spangenberg, E. R., & Greenwald, A. G. (1999). Social influence by requesting self-prophecy. Journal of Consumer Psychology, 8, 61-89.

6. Huang, K., Yeomans, M., Brooks, A. W., Minson, J., & Gino, F. (2017). It doesn't hurt to ask: Question-asking increases liking. Journal of Personality and Social Psychology, 113(3), 430–452. https://doi.org/10.1037/pspi0000097

7. The kiss of the porcupines: From attributing responsibility to forgiving FRANK D. FINCHAM. Personal Relationships, 7 (2000), 1-23.

12 *The Good Feud Guide*

1. Mental health consequences of minority political positions: The case of Brexit. Social Science & Medicine. Christopher W. N. Saville Volume 258, August 2020, 113016.
2. Interruptions in political interviews: a study of Margaret Thatcher and Neil Kinnock Peter Bull and Kate Mayer, Journal of Language and Social Psychology
3. Farley, S. D. (2008). Attaining status at the expense of likeability: Pilfering power through conversational interruption. Journal of Nonverbal Behavior, 32, 241–260.
4. James, D., & Clarke, S. (1993). Women, men, and interruptions: A critical review. In D. Tannen (Ed.), Gender and conversational interaction (pp. 231–280). New York, NY: Oxford University Press.
5. Effects of Sex of Subject, Sex of Interrupter, and Topic of Conversation on the Perceptions of Interruptions Catherine A. Chambliss, Norah Feeny First Published December 1, 1992 Research Article https://doi.org/10.2466/pms.1992.75.3f.1235
6. Does Frequency of Interruptions Amplify the Effect of Various Types of Interruptions? Experimental Evidence Augusto Gnisci, Ida Sergi, Elvira De Luca Vanessa Errico Journal of Nonverbal Behavior volume 36, pages39–57(2012) 355
7. The strategy of psychopathy: primary psychopathic traits predict defection on low-value relationships Matthew M. Gervais,1,2 Michelle Kline,1,2 Mara Ludmer,1 Rachel George,1,3 and Joseph H. Manson1, Proc Biol Sci. 2013 Apr 22; 280(1757): 20122773. doi: 10.1098/rspb.2012.2773 PMCID: PMC3619474 PMID: 23446522
8. Roy F. Baumeister, Kathleen D. Vohs, Jennifer L. Aaker & Emily N. Garbinsky (2013) Some key differences between a happy life and a meaningful life, The Journal of Positive Psychology, 8:6, 505-516, DOI: 10.1080/17439760.2013.830764 http://dx.doi.org/10.1080/17439760.2013.830764
9. Horowitz, M., and S. Meffert. "Revenge Fantasies." (2007): 391-394. Encyclopaedia of Stress Hardcover ISBN: 9780120885039 Imprint: Academic Press Published Date: 8th May 2007
   Mardi J. Horowitz. Understanding and Ameliorating Revenge Fantasies in Psychotherapy. The American Journal of Psychiatry, Volume 164, Issue 1, January, 2007, Pages 24-27
10. Casey Ryan Kelly (2020). Donald J. Trump and the rhetoric of ressentiment. Quarterly Journal of Speech. 106:1, 2-24
11. Peter Strelan, Jan-Willem Van Prooijen and Mario Gollwitzer (2019). When transgressors intend to cause harm: The empowering effects of revenge and forgiveness on victim well-being. British Journal of Social Psychology (2019). 59(2)
12. Knoll, J. L. IV. (2010). The 'pseudocommando' mass murderer: Part 1: The psychology of revenge and obliteration. Journal of the American Academy of Psychiatry and the Law, 38(1), 87–94.

Notes

13 *Inside the Minds of Those Trolling Captain Sir Tom Moore*

1. Death and Lulz: Understanding the personality characteristics of RIP trolls by Kathryn C. Seigfried-Spellar and Siddharth S. Chowdhury. First Monday, Volume 22, Number 11 – 6 November 2017 https://journals.uic.edu/ojs/index.php/fm/article/download/7861/6556 doi: http://dx.doi.org/10.5210/fm.v22i11.7861
2. Appreciation of achievement and a behavioural preference to view failure: Schadenfreude online. James Phillips, Erik Landhuis, Jay Wood. Personality and Individual Differences Volume 172, April 2021, 110597

14 *Coping with Quarantine*

1. Andhra Pradesh: Man ends life relating his fever to Coronavirus https://punemirror.indiatimes.com/news/india/andhra-pradesh-man-ends-life-relating-his-fever-to-corona-virus/articleshow/74088283.cms?utm_source=contentofinterest&utm_medium=text&utm_campaign=cppst
2. The psychological impact of quarantine and how to reduce it: rapid review of the evidence. Samantha K Brooks, Rebecca K Webster, Louise Smith, Lisa Woodland, Simon Wessely, Neil Greenberg, Gideon James Rubin. The Lancet, Published: February 26, 2020 DOI:https://doi.org/10.1016/S0140-6736(20)30460-8
3. Tapei Times Sun, Apr 19, 2020 page8 Taiwan in Time: Remembering the SARS lockdown. Panic ensued as the ill-prepared Hoping Hospital was sealed off on April 24, 2003 with more than 1,000 people inside after a suspected cluster infection. By Han Cheung / Staff reporter
4. Is There a Case for Quarantine? Perspectives from SARS to Ebola. Donna Barbisch, Kristi Koenig and Fuh-Yuan Shih. Disaster medicine and public health preparedness, Volume 9, Issue 5 October 2015, pp. 547-553.
5. Factors influencing psychological distress during a disease epidemic: Data from Australia's first out-break of equine influenza. Melanie Taylor, Kingsley Agho, Garry Stevens & Beverley Raphael. BMC Public Health volume 8, Article number: 347 (2008)
6. Parenthood and Host Resistance to the Common Cold. Rodlescia Sneed, Sheldon Cohen, Donald Turner and William Doyle. Psychosomatic Medicine. 2012 Jul-Aug; 74(6): 567–573.doi: 10.1097/PSY.0b013e31825941ff
7. The Psychology of Coping With Quarantine https://www.psychologytoday.com/gb/blog/slightly-blighty/202003/the-psychology-coping-quarantine

15 *Does Lockdown Inflict the Same Mental Health Effects as Imprisonment??*

1. Are People Experiencing the 'Pains of Imprisonment' During the COVID-19 Lockdown? Mandeep K. Dhami, Leonardo Weiss-Cohen and Peter Ayton. Front. Psychol., 19 November 2020 https://doi.org/10.3389/fpsyg.2020.578430
2. Economic suicides in the Great Recession in Europe and North America Aaron Reeves, Martin McKee and David Stuckler. British Journal of Psychiatry. Volume 205, Issue 3 September 2014, pp. 246-247

3. Weems, C. F., Carrion, V. G., McCurdy, B. H., and Scozzafava, M. D. (2020). Increased Risk of Suicide due to Economic and Social Impacts of Social Distancing Measures to Address the COVID-19 Pandemic: A Forecast. Available online at: https://www.researchgate.net/publication/340487993 (accessed June 29, 2020).

16 Psychologists Predict Public Rebellion Will Erupt against the Lockdown

1. American faces prison in Thailand over bad hotel review. Wesley Barnes sued by resort owner after posting negative comments on Tripadvisor. https://www.theguardian.com/world/2020/sep/29/american-wesley-barnes-faces-prison-thailand-bad-hotel-review
   https://www.tripadvisor.co.uk/Hotel_Review-g580110-d594766-Reviews-Sea_View_Resort_Spa_Koh_Chang-Ko_Chang_Trat_Province.html
2. Milgram S (1963) Behavioral study of obedience. Journal of Abnormal and Social Psychology, 67: 371–378.
   Milgram S (1974) Obedience to Authority: An Experimental View. Harper Collins.
3. Haslam A, Reicher SD (2017): 50 years of 'obedience to authority': from blind conformity to engaged followership. Annual Review of Law and Social Science, 13: 59–78.
4. In their approach to coronavirus lockdown, our leaders may have made a fundamental mistake about human psychology https://inews.co.uk/opinion/coronavirus-lockdown-psychology-misunderstanding-417533
5. A fall in autumn: Why Europe's second, less severe lockdowns are working. The restrictions have limited the rate of new infections, especially from long trips. https://www.economist.com/graphic-detail/2020/11/28/why-europes-second-less-severe-lockdowns-are-working

17 Can Dominic Cummings' Mindset Explain Lockdown Laxity?

1. Top officials around the world keep getting caught breaking lockdown rules By Siobhán O'Grady Staff Writer, Foreign desk May 26, 2020 at 6:00 a.m. GMT+1 www.washingtonpost.com/world/2020/05/06/top-officials-around-world-keep-getting-caught-breaking-lockdown-rules/
2. Boris Johnson faces renewed Tory pressure to sack Dominic Cummings Rowena Mason Deputy political editor Mon 25 May 2020 14.36 BST The Guardian https://www.theguardian.com/politics/2020/may/25/boris-johnson-faces-renewed-tory-pressure-to-sack-dominic-cummings
3. On either side of a moat? Elite and mass attitudes towards right and wrong. Nicholas Allen & Sarah Birch European Journal of Political Research 51: 89–116, 2012
4. Schlenker BR, Pontari BA, Christopher AN. Excuses and Character: Personal and Social Implications of Excuses. Personality and Social Psychology Review. 2001;5(1):15-32. doi:10.1207/S15327957PSPR0501_2
5. Can Dominic Cummings Psychology Explain Lockdown Violations? https://www.psychologytoday.com/gb/blog/slightly-blighty/202005/can-dominic-cummings-psychology-explain-lockdown-violations

18 The Psychology behind Neil Ferguson's Resignation Scandal

1. How Neil Ferguson, the architect of lockdown, was brought down by failing to obey his own rules Government's leading epidemiology adviser set out advice that led to UK restrictions in research paper submitted on March 16 ByAnna Mikhailova, deputy political editor; Christopher Hope, chief political correspondent; Louisa Wells and Michael Gillard5 May 2020 • 9:02pm The Daily Telegraph https://www.telegraph.co.uk/news/2020/05/05/neil-ferguson-architect-lockdown-brought-failing-obey-rules/

2. Professor Neil Ferguson had to go but Sage will be a lesser body without him. History will be kind to Prof Ferguson, his 'suppression' strategy came too late for the UK economy but saved thousands of lives By Paul Nuki, global health security editor, London 6 May 2020 • 8:58pm The Daily Telegraph https://www.telegraph.co.uk/global-health/science-and-disease/had-go-sage-will-lesser-body-without/

3. Teaching may be hazardous to your marriage Satoshi Kanazawaa, Mary Still. Evolution and Human Behavior 21 (2000) 185–190

4. One woman's behavior affects the attractiveness of others. Sandeep Mishra, Andrew Clark, Martin Daly. Evolution and Human Behavior 28 (2007) 145 – 149

5. The Psychology Behind the UK Government Adviser's Resignation Scandal https://www.psychologytoday.com/gb/blog/slightly-blighty/202005/the-psychology-behind-the-uk-government-advisers-resignation-scandal

19 Did COVID Karma Kill Trump's Campaign?

1. Most Americans say Trump acted irresponsibly and distrust White House on his health. By Jennifer Agiesta, CNN Polling Director Updated 2344 GMT (0744 HKT) October 5, 2020. https://edition.cnn.com/2020/10/05/politics/cnn-poll-coronavirus-trump/index.html

2. 'She Doesn't Have the Stamina': Hillary Clinton and the Hysteria Diagnosis in the 2016 Presidential Election. Ryan Neville-Shepard &Jaclyn Nolan Pages 60-79 | Published online: 10 May 2019. Women's Studies in Communication Volume 42, 2019 — Issue 1

3. The Mortal Presidency: Illness and Anguish in the White House. Robert Gilbert. Fordham University Press; 2Rev Ed Edition (28 Feb. 1998)

4. The health of the President and presidential candidates: the public's right to know. G J Annas. N Engl J Med. 1995 Oct 5;333(14):945-9. doi: 10.1056/NEJM199510053331420

5. The right look: Conservative politicians look better and voters reward it Niclas Berggren Henrik Jordahl Panu Poutvaar *Journal of Public Economics* Volume 146, February 2017, Pages 79-86

6. Why are right wing voters attracted to to dominant leaders? Assessing competing theories of psychological mechanisms Lasse Laustsen Michael Bang Petersen The Leadership Quarterly Volume 31, Issue 2, April 2020, 101301

7. Election systems, the 'beauty premium' in politics, and the beauty of dissent European Journal of Political Economy Niklas Potrafke Marcus Rösch Heinrich Ursprung Volume 64, September 2020, 101900

8. The Captive King and His Captive Court: The Psychopolitical Dynamics of the Disabled Leader and His Inner Circle. Jerrold M. Post, Robert S. Robins. Political Psychology, 1990, 11 (2), 331-351

The Captive King and His Captive Court: The Psychopolitical Dynamics of the Disabled Leader and His Inner Circle. Jerrold M. Post, Robert S. Robins. Family Business Review, vol. VI, no. 2, Summer 1993

9. When Illness Strikes the Leader: The Dilemma of the Captive King. Jerrold M. Post, Robert S. Robins. New Haven, CT: Yale University Press, 1993, 320 pp. US$25.00 cloth. ISBN 0-300-05683-4. Yale University Press, 302 Temple St., New Haven, CT 06511, USA.

10. Did Winston Churchill suffer a myocardial infarction in the White House at Christmas 1941? J Allister Vale, John W Scadding. Journal of the Royal Society of Medicine Vol 110, Issue 12, 2017

11. Facial Cues to Perceived Height Influence Leadership Choices in Simulated War and Peace Contexts. Daniel E. Re, Lisa M. DeBruine, Benedict C. Jones. Evolutionary Psychology, Volume: 11 issue: 1. January 1, 2013

12. Could COVID Karma Kill Trump's Campaign? www.psychologytoday.com/gb/blog/slightly-blighty/202010/could-covid-karma-kill-trumps-campaign

13. The Mental Impact of Boris Johnson's Hospitalization https://www.psychologytoday.com/gb/blog/slightly-blighty/202004/the-mental-impact-boris-johnsons-hospitalization

20 Does the Pandemic Mean that the Future Is Now Female?

1. Garikipati, Supriya and Kambhampati, Uma, Leading the Fight Against the Pandemic: Does Gender 'Really' Matter? (June 3, 2020). Available at SSRN: https://ssrn.com/abstract=3617953 or http://dx.doi.org/10.2139/ssrn.3617953

2. Potential lessons from the Taiwan and New Zealand health responses to the COVID-19 pandemic Dr Jennifer Summers Dr Hao-Yuan Cheng Professor Hsien-Ho Lin Dr Lucy Telfar Barnard Dr Amanda Kvalsvig Professor Nick Wilson Professor Michael G Baker The Lancet Regional Health West Pacific VOLUME 4, 100044, NOVEMBER 01, 2020 Published: October 21, 2020DOI:https://doi.org/10.1016/j.lanwpc.2020.100044

3. Why do female leaders seem so good at tackling the coronavirus pandemic? By Jennifer Rigby, Sarah Newey and Dominic Gilbert 28 April 2020 • 6:00am The Daily Telegraph https://www.telegraph.co.uk/global-health/science-and-disease/do-female-leaders-seem-good-tackling-coronavirus-pandemic/

4. What Do Countries With The Best Coronavirus Responses Have In Common? Women Leaders Avivah Wittenberg-Cox https://www.forbes.com/sites/avivahwittenbergcox/2020/04/13/what-do-Forbes Magazine countries-with-the-best-coronavirus-reponses-have-in-common-women-leaders/?sh=63fca6b63dec

5. #wearetogether: female led countries' covid-19 outcomes 'systematically and significantly better' https://www.reading.ac.uk/news-and-events/releases/PR846481.aspx

6. Getting on top of the glass cliff: Reviewing a decade of evidence, explanations, and impact Michelle K Ryan a S. Alexander Haslam Thekla Morgenroth FloorRink Janka Stoker Kim Peters The Leadership Quarterly Volume 27, Issue 3, June 2016, Pages 446-455

7. Gender, Violence, and International Crisis Mary Caprioli, Mark A. Boyer First Published August 1, 2001 https://doi.org/10.1177/0022002701045004005 Vol 45, Issue 4, 2001 Journal of Conflict Resolution.

8. Personality and Individual Differences Volume 33, Issue 5, 5 October 2002, Pages 803-813 Feminine values and happy life-expectancy in nations W.Aarrindell RVeenhoven

9. Do Female Presidents or Prime Ministers Make Any Difference? Research finds 'feminine' values make a difference. But do female leaders? Posted Jul 09, 2016 Psychology Today Raj Persaud, M.D. and Peter Bruggen, M.D. Slightly Blighty www.psychologytoday.com/gb/blog/slightly-blighty/201607/do-female-presidents-or-prime-ministers-make-any-difference

10. Why Women Make Better Crisis Leaders https://www.project-syndicate.org/commentary/woman-leaders-covid-19-crisis-ardern-by-raj-persaud-2020-05?barrier=accesspaylog

21 *Will COVID Stress Have an Impact on Future Generations?*

1. Family Ruptures, Stress, and the Mental Health of the Next Generation. Petra Persson and Maya Rossin-Slater American Economic Review 2018, 108(4-5): 1214–1252 https://doi.org/10.1257/aer.20141406

2. Black, Sandra E., Paul J. Devereux, and Kjell G. Salvanes. 2016. 'Does Grief Transfer Across Generations' Applied Economics 8(1):193–223.

3. R.G. Gitau, A. Cameron, N.M. Fisk, V. Glover Fetal exposure to maternal cortisol Lancet, 352 (1998), pp. 707-708

4. Malaspina, D., Corcoran, C., Kleinhaus, K. et al. Acute maternal stress in pregnancy and schizophrenia in offspring: A cohort prospective study. BMC Psychiatry 8, 71 (2008). https://doi.org/10.1186/1471-244X-8-71

5. Brown AS, Begg MD, Gravenstein S, et al. Serologic Evidence of Prenatal Influenza in the Etiology of Schizophrenia. Arch Gen Psychiatry. 2004;61(8):774–780. doi:10.1001/archpsyc.61.8.774

6. Garthwaite, Craig. 2008. 'The Effect of In-Utero Conditions on Long Term Health: Evidence from the 1918 Spanish Flu Pandemic.' Available at http://www.kellogg.northwestern.edu/faculty/garthwaite/htm/fetal_stress_garthwaite_053008.pdf

7. Does in utero exposure to Illness matter? The 1918 influenza epidemic in Taiwan as a natural experiment. Ming-Jen Lin, Elaine M. Liub. Journal of Health Economics, Volume 37, September 2014, Pages 152-163

8. It's Just a Game The Super Bowl and Low Birth Weight. Duncan, Brian; Mansour, Hani; Rees, Daniel I. Journal of Human Resources. Fall 2017, Vol. 52 Issue 4, p946-978. 33p. DOI: 10.3368/jhr.52.4.0615-7213R.

9. Richter, A., & Robling, P. O. (2013). Multigenerational effects of the 1918–19 influenza pandemic in Sweden (Working Paper 5/2013). Stockholm, Sweden: Swedish Institute for Social Research, Stockholm University.

Richter, A., & Robling, P. O. (2015). Multigenerational effects of the 1918–19 influenza pandemic on educational attainment: Evidence from Sweden. In P. O. Robling (Ed.), Essays on the origins of human capital, crime and income inequality (p. 16). Stockholm, Sweden: Swedish Institute for Social Research, Stockholm University.

10. Epidemics and Trust: The Case of the Spanish Flu Arnstein Aassve, Guido Alfani, Francesco Gandolfi, Marco Le Moglie. Working Paper n. 661 This Version: March, 2020 IGIER – Università Bocconi, Via Guglielmo Röntgen 1, 20136 Milano – Italy http://www.igier.unibocconi.it

    Aassve, A., Alfani, G., Gandolfi, F. and Le Moglie, M. (2021), Epidemics and trust: The case of the Spanish Flu. Health Economics. https://doi.org/10.1002/hec.4218

11. Can COVID-19 Stress Have an Impact on Pregnancy? The scientific literature on pregnancy stress and later psychological problems Posted May 05, 2020 www.psychologytoday.com/gb/blog/slightly-blighty/202005/can-covid-19-stress-have-impact-pregnancy

22 What Happens If There Are No Doctors?

1. Being Mortal Illness, medicine and what matters in the end Atul Gawande 1 July 2015 304pp ISBN 9781846685828
2. Lance Armstrong, It's Not about the Bike: My Journey Back to Life. Yellow Jersey Press 2001 ISBN 10: 0224060872 – ISBN 13: 9780224060875
3. Cunningham S A, Mitchell K et al. Doctors' strikes and mortality: a review. Soc Sci Med 2008;67:1784-1788
4. Jena AB, Prasad V, Goldman DP, Romley J. Mortality and Treatment Patterns Among Patients Hospitalized With Acute Cardiovascular Conditions During Dates of National Cardiology Meetings. JAMA Intern Med. 2015;175(2):237–244. doi:10.1001/jamainternmed.2014.6781
5. Is Survival After Out-of-Hospital Cardiac Arrests Worse During Days of National Academic Meetings in Japan? A Population-Based Study. Tetsuhisa Kitamura, Kosuke Kiyohara, Tasuku Matsuyama, Toshihiro Hatakeyama, Tomonari Shimamoto, Junichi Izawa, Chika Nishiyama, Taku Iwami Journal of Epidemiology Volume 26 (2016) Issue 3

23 Can Pandemic Paranoia Produce Mass Killing?

1. Jedwab, Remi, Noel D. Johnson, and Mark Koyama. 'Negative shocks and mass persecutions: evidence from the Black Death.' Journal of Economic Growth 24.4 (2019): 345-395.
2. 'Do Natural Disasters Enhance Societal Trust?' Mark Skidmore and Hideki Toya, Kyklos, Vol 67 (2), 2014.
3. Moscow is accused of hiding military spies among a group of doctors it had sent to Italy's coronavirus epicentre. By Jack Wright For Mailonline Published: 19:37, 3 April 2020 | UPDATED: 19:58, 3 April 2020 https://www.dailymail.co.uk/news/article-8185677/Moscow-accused-hiding-military-spies-doctors-sent-Italys-coronavirus-epicentre.html

4. Persecution & Toleration: The Long Road to Religious Freedom (Cambridge Studies in Economics, Choice, and Society) Noel D. Johnson, and Mark Koyama Cambridge University Press 2019
5. Can Pandemic Paranoia Produce Mass Murder? Research explores how pandemics and other catastrophes can drive us to war www.psychologytoday.com/gb/blog/slightly-blighty/202004/can-pandemic-paranoia-produce-mass-murder

24 Does Fighting COVID on the Streets Need a New Churchill?

1. Can Churchill's Speech Psychology Explain Oscar Success? Gary Oldman and the film Darkest Hour owe their success to speech inspiration www.psychologytoday.com/gb/blog/slightly-blighty/201803/can-churchill-s-speech-psychology-explain-oscar-success
2. The Influence of a Simulated 'Pep Talk' on Athlete Inspiration, Situational Motivation, and Emotion. Stephen P. Gonzalez, Jonathan N. Metzler and Maria Newton. International Journal of Sports Science & Coaching Volume 6 · Number 3, 2011
3. Power motivation, activation, and inspirational speeches. Robert S. Steele. Journal of Personality. Volume 45, Issue 1, March 1977, Pages 53–64
4. Inspiration as a Psychological Construct. Todd M. Thrash and Andrew J. Elliot. Journal of Personality and Social Psychology. 2003, Vol. 84, No. 4, 871–889
5. The Mantle of the Prophet: Churchill's Embodiment of the Prophetic Ethos. Andrew Bowman. Young Scholars in Writing. 2015
6. Presidential leadership and charisma: The effects of metaphor. Jeffery Scott Mio, Ronald E.Riggio, Shana Levin, Renford Reese. The Leadership Quarterly. Volume 16, Issue 2, April 2005, Pages 287-294
7. Admiration for virtue: Neuroscientific perspectives on a motivating emotion Contemporary Educational Psychology, Volume 35, Issue 2, April 2010, Pages 110-115 Mary Helen Immordino-Yang, Lesley Sylvan

25 The 'Boomerang' Effect of Vaccinating three Former US Presidents

1. Obama, Clinton and Bush pledge to take Covid vaccine on TV to show its safety Adam Gabbatt @adamgabbatt Thu 3 Dec 2020 16.18 GMT https://www.theguardian.com/us-news/2020/dec/03/obama-clinton-bush-covid-vaccine-safety
2. Clinical Outcomes Of A COVID-19 Vaccine: Implementation Over Efficacy A. David Paltiel, Jason L. Schwartz, Amy Zheng, and Rochelle P. Walensky. Health Affairs ahead of print. Published November 19, 2020 https://doi.org/10.1377/hlthaff.2020.02054
3. Government Health Warnings and the "Boomerang" Effect. Michael Hyland, James Birrell. Psychological Reports Vol 44, Issue 2, 1979 First Published April 1, 1979 Research Article Find in PubMed https://doi.org/10.2466/pro.1979.44.2.643
4. Are Graphic Cigarette Warning Labels an Effective Message Strategy? A Test of Psychological Reactance Theory and Source Appraisal Nicole R. LaVoie, Brian L. Quick, Julius M. Riles and Natalie J. Lambert. Communication Research 2017, Vol. 44(3) 416–436

5. Aharon Levy & Yossi Maaravi (2018) The boomerang effect of psychological interventions. Social Influence, 13:1, 39-51, DOI: 10.1080/15534510.2017.1421571
6. Populist politics and vaccine hesitancy in Western Europe: an analysis of national-level data Jonathan Kennedy European Journal of Public Health, Volume 29, Issue 3, June 2019, Pages 512–516, https://doi.org/10.1093/eurpub/ckz004

26 COVID on the Couch: Sigmund Freud's Surprising Analysis
1. Recommendations for Psychoanalysts Regarding the Use of Videoconferencing in their Practice. International Psychoanalytical Association. https://www.ipa.world/IPA/en/News/corona_remote_sessions.aspx
2. Therapy Under Lockdown – I'm just as terrified as my patients are. Gary Greenberg. The Guardian Newspaper April 23 https://www.theguardian.com/society/2020/apr/23/therapy-during-coronavirus-pandemic-lockdown-psychoanalysis-freud
3. Age-Specific Mortality During the 1918 Influenza Pandemic: Unravelling the Mystery of High Young Adult Mortality. Alain Gagnon, Matthew S. Miller, Stacey A. Hallman, Robert Bourbeau, D. Ann Herring, David JD. Earn, Joaquín Madrenas. PLOS One https://doi.org/10.1371/journal.pone.0069586
   Pandemic Paradox: Early Life H2N2 Pandemic Influenza Infection Enhanced Susceptibility to Death during the 2009 H1N1 Pandemic Alain Gagnon, Enrique Acosta, Stacey Hallman, Robert Bourbeau, Lisa Y. Dillon, Nadine Ouellette, David J. D. Earn, D. Ann Herring, Kris Inwood, Joaquin Madrenas, Matthew S. Miller mBio Jan 2018, 9 (1) e02091-17; DOI: 10.1128/mBio.02091-17
4. Letter from Sigmund Freud to Oskar Pfister, January 27, 1920. Psychoanalytic Electronic Publishing https://www.pep-web.org/document.php?id=zbk.051.0327a
5. Psychoanalysis and Faith: The Letters of Sigmund Freud and Oskar Pfister, eds. Heinrich Meng and Ernst L. Freud, trans. by Eric Mosbacher. New York: Basic Books, 1963 (or elsewhere I saw 1964).
6. Freud: A Very Short Introduction (Very Short Introductions) Paperback – 22 Feb. 2001. Anthony Storr. Oxford University Press
7. Psychoanalysis and Faith: Sigmund Freud and Oskar Pfister (Book Review) Storr, Anthony. New Society; London Vol. 2, Iss. 62, (Dec 5, 1963): 25.
8. COVID-19 on the Couch: Sigmund Freud's Surprising Analysis. What would the founder of psychoanalysis, Sigmund Freud, say today about coping? Posted Apr 26, 2020 https://www.psychologytoday.com/gb/blog/slightly-blighty/202004/covid-19-the-couch-sigmund-freuds-surprising-analysis
9. Letter from Freud to Ludwig Binswanger, April 11, 1929. Psychoanalytic Electronic Publishing. http://www.pep-web.org/document.php?id=zbk.050.0196a

Epilogue
1. Suicide in the Media: A Quantitative Review of Studies Based on Nonfictional Stories. Steven Stack. Suicide and Life-Threatening Behavior 35(2) April 2005, 121-133
2. Internet Searches for Suicide Following the Release of 13 Reasons Why. Ayers JW, Althouse BM, Leas EC, Dredze M, Allem J. JAMA Intern Med. 2017;177(10):1527–1529. doi:10.1001/jamainternmed.2017.3333

3. Association between the release of Netflix's 13 Reasons Why and suicide rates in the United States: an interrupted times series analysis. Bridge, J, Greenhouse, JB, Ruch, D, Stevens, J, Ackerman, J, Sheftall, A, et al. J Am Acad Child Adolesc Psychiatry 2019; 28 Apr (doi: 10.1016/j.jaac.2019.04.020).

4. Fink DS, Santaella-Tenorio J and Keyes KM (2018) Increase in suicides the months after the death of Robin Williams in the US. PLoS ONE 13: e0191405.

5. Role of media reports in completed and prevented suicide: Werther v. Papageno effects. Thomas Niederkrotenthaler, Martin Voracek, Arno Herberth, Benedikt Till, Markus Strauss, Elmar Etzersdorfer, Brigitte Eisenwort and Gernot Sonneck. British Journal of Psychiatry, 197(3), 234-243. doi:10.1192/bjp.bp.109.074633

6. What the highest rated movie of all time may teach us about portraying suicide in film Mark Sinyor, Steven Stack and Thomas Niederkrotenthaler. Australian & New Zealand Journal of Psychiatry 2020, Vol. 54(3) 223–224

7. Patterdale mountain rescue of volunteer 'worst in 25 years' Published16 February Patterdale mountain rescue of volunteer 'worst in 25 years' Published16 February BBC News
   Mountain rescuer who fell 500ft trying to help lockdown flouters will be in a wheelchair for life By Gareth Davies, 16 February 2021 • 12:08pm The Daily Telegraph https://www.telegraph.co.uk/news/2021/02/16/mountain-rescuer-fell-500ft-trying-help-lockdown-flouters-will/

8. Emperor Hirohito, Accepting the Potsdam Declaration, Radio Broadcast.
   Transmitted by Domei and Recorded by the Federal Communications Commission, 14 August 1945 https://www.mtholyoke.edu/acad/intrel/hirohito.htm

9. The Emperor's Speech: 67 Years Ago, Hirohito Transformed Japan Forever
   Max Fisher August 15, 2012 The Atlantic https://www.theatlantic.com/international/archive/2012/08/the-emperors-speech-67-years-ago-hirohito-transformed-japan-forever/261166/

10. 14th August 2020 VJ Day: This is how Japan surrendered to save its emperor
    By Martin Hannan The National https://www.thenational.scot/news/18650176.vj-day-japan-surrendered-save-emperor/